Nature's Hidden Oracles

LIZ DEAN

For Michael Young

An Hachette UK Company www.hachette.co.uk

First published in Great Britain in 2021 by Godsfield, an imprint of
Octopus Publishing Group Ltd
Carmelite House
50 Victoria Embankment, London EC4Y 0DZ
www.octopusbooks.co.uk

Distributed in the US by Hachette Book Group
1290 Avenue of the Americas,
4th and 5th Floors, New York, NY 10104

Distributed in Canada by Canadian Manda Group
664 Annette St., Toronto, Ontario, Canada M6S 2C8

ISBN 978 1 84181 494 0
A CIP catalogue record for this book is available from
the British Library.

Printed and bound in China
10 9 8 7 6 5 4 3

Publishing Director: Stephanie Jackson
Senior Managing Editor: Sybella Stephens
Designer: Jack Storey
Illustrator: Celia Hart
Senior Production Controller: Emily Noto

Nature's Hidden Oracles

From flowers to feathers &
shells to stones – a practical
guide to natural divination

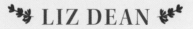 **LIZ DEAN**

With illustrations by Celia Hart

GODSFIELD

Contents

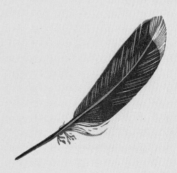

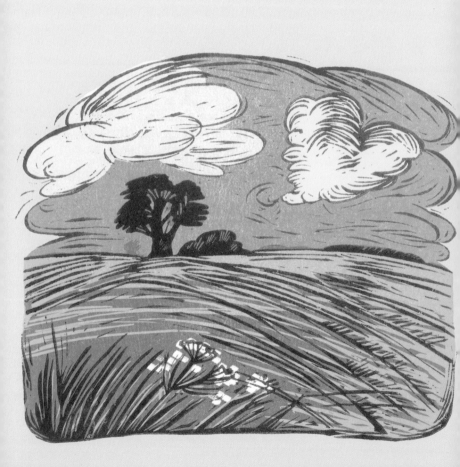

The natural connection

Introduction

Nature's Hidden Oracles is an invitation to reconnect with nature and with yourself. When you are peaceful and connected with the natural world, you feel at one with yourself, and the natural world – and can intuit whatever guidance you need. These tools of insight that exist within and arise from nature – and which we call oracles – offer creative ways to approach life, and to see yourself and your story spelled out within the natural world – in wood, stone, seashells, feathers, flowers and herbs.

Oracular divination is the seeking of advice or hidden knowledge from the gods, or the "divine". When you divine in nature, you're working openly using what is available around you, from interpreting clouds to reading ripples in water or patterns in sand. Those of you who are already divining with cards, tea leaves or other tools may find that casting oracles outdoors feels very different from giving readings inside. It's freeing and creative – and takes us all out of smaller, darker spaces into the wider natural world, to be seen.

Receptive & active divination

Roman augurs, or official diviners, saw divination in two ways: as messages received in answer to a question and as messages received by chance. So, one is deliberate: holding an intention – or consciously deciding – to find an answer or insight about a situation and waiting for an answer; and the other is seeing a sign you didn't consciously ask for. Much Roman augury focused on interpreting the flights of birds and the weather to see if the gods were for or against a course of action, rather than actively divining, hands on, using natural materials to hand. However, this is where, and how, we begin – with slow walking or standing or sitting still for long enough to notice a sign; being open to what nature will do; being willing to receive.

When you can receive by looking at what's around you – seeing forms and patterns in the landscape (see overleaf), you're ready to become more active, to get into reading the detail on a tree trunk, the petals on a flower; to choose and cast stones on the beach or collect your own oracle twigs (see Chapter 1, pages 48–55) or natural charms (see Chapter 5, pages 130–9).

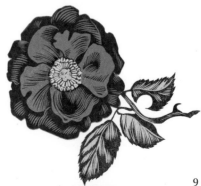

Techniques

You may not need techniques at all. For some, being in nature is enough to switch on their oracular radar. After all, outdoor divination can be second nature – just a step along from blowing a dandelion clock or picking those daisy petals for yes or no. However, techniques can help when your mind is over-busy, because they offer a structured focus that shifts you away from unwanted thoughts. The techniques given here get you into a divinatory space and help keep you there, immersed.

How to ask a question

The rituals in this book assume that you'll be reading for yourself, asking questions about your past, present and future, or giving a reading to a friend. You may also feel called to ask broader questions – about the environment, for example, or about the area you choose for your divination. You might ask the land what it has to say. You may discover you have a bond with a place in nature that's special to you, and want to investigate this in a reading. When asking about people in your life, don't ask about their secrets, but do ask how their behaviour or character might impact upon you, if this is a key issue. And it's fine not to have a question in mind; you can simply begin divining, trusting that you'll find the guidance and ideas you need as you go along.

Sometimes, the first questions that come to mind may not be the ones you need to ask. There's no such thing as the wrong question, but you can get so used to asking yourself the same thing from day to day that you may not realize that the question needs to change. Also, if you have a hard agenda, seeking the answer to one big question, it sets up a block in your reading. You may find it hard to connect because you're running ahead into the future, into the ideal outcome. If this is the case, let go of the wanting – replace your fear with trust that you will gain the insights and answers you need. Be open to what might happen, to the unexpected, and change the question if you need to.

Asking a question in divination is rather like finding the right key to a lock. Try the meditation on the following page and see what happens – if your original question or issue comes back, it's confirmation that it still needs to be asked or dealt with. If you sense a different question, go with it.

Connect with nature

Finding the right space to relax and connect with nature (see page 15) helps us ask the right questions of our oracles. When you are comfortable and ready to do your divination, take a deep breath in and out, and feel your physical connection with the earth through your feet. This brings you into the present moment. Take your attention to your breathing and let your senses open up to the environment. If thoughts are getting in the way, visualize a box and place your worries and stress inside it. Take the box and rest it on a shelf to your left-hand side.

Everything is perfect.

All is well.

Now, feel the space inside your body – visualize this as a light under your rib cage that gets bigger and brighter every time you breathe in and out. Wait for your question, or the subject of your enquiry, to come to you, like a fish flipping up from a still pool.

How to receive information and know it's real

When you are reading oracles in nature, go with your first impression. When you're relaxed and centred during divination, the first thought that comes in is your intuition. It lands in a flash, as a knowing, an instant truth. If you don't recognize it as intuition, or doubt it, it is quickly overlapped by thoughts that are your programming – the things you are used to thinking. It's a kind of running script, a reflex that doesn't feel quite right. So speak your intuitive impression right away. It's rather like remembering a dream – just as you're waking up you see an image, then try to hold on to it, but the harder you try the more it disappears, out of reach. The key is not to try, not to over-think. Just say instantly what you feel and see, and you'll find this opens a doorway to intuitive information. You may find yourself speaking without knowing why; you may sense a colour or see an image in your mind that feels true. Trust this first impression, and go with it. Doing so may feel like a leap of faith, and it is. Intuitive thoughts may be described as flashes, but they are often subtle and come quietly, without any emotional charge. Catch them when you can.

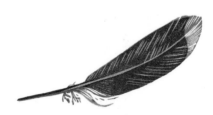

Being in nature helps you notice subtle intuitive messages, because your senses are already switched on, attuned to the natural environment. If you doubt your intuitive knowing, this blocks you and makes you feel disconnected. If this happens to you, use touch to get reconnected – feel the indentations in bark, run your fingers through grass. The more you practise divination in nature, the easier it becomes to identify, trust and speak your first impression as soon as you begin a reading.

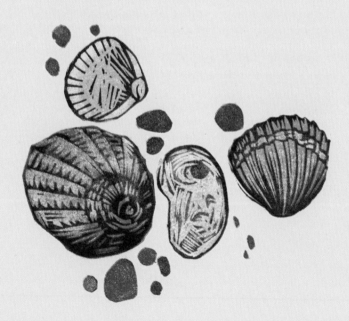

Finding space

Before you begin working with the oracles in this book, find a place for yourself within nature: sit with your back against a tree trunk, lie down and bathe in the forest (see Forest Bathing on page 27) or wander into the grass. When we enter wild places, we're reconnecting with a part of us that is natural, too – the self that is not stressed, or longing for something, or dissatisfied. The part of us that wants to create, to join in. Having physical space creates space in our mind to receive insights and messages. Out in nature, we become more sensitive, more aware of our surroundings and our responses. We become our true selves. We see hidden symbols, signs, patterns; we make meaning – and become insight-seers rather than sightseers.

Using this book

I have at times given lists of meanings – for symbol shapes, the number of petals found on a flower, feather colours and types of herb, for example. These listings are not intended to replace your own knowing, but to help you build a reading if divination is new to you. With practice you won't need them. But in the beginning they will help you connect with nature, hopefully inspiring your imagination and creativity. Most of the oracles in the book have you look at different aspects of your life, often with reference to the past, present or future. In this context, "future" or "outcome" means the most likely outcome given the present circumstances. It is not destiny; a reading is a glimpse ahead, to what might happen should things continue as they are. At any point you may make a decision that alters this potential outcome. This is also relevant to the "yes/no" readings; again, the answer reflects the moment and may change if you repeat it later.

Keeping a journal

You might like to photograph the signs you see and the oracles you cast while you're out and about. If you prefer to go into nature without technology, take a notebook with you and write down or draw your findings. Add the date, and you'll appreciate looking back over your nature notes in the weeks and months to come.

Reading together

You will see that I recommend working with a friend for some of the rituals. Having a walking companion or a small group of companions empowers your readings. You can read for each other, of course, but it's very helpful, too, when reading for yourself. When a friend or two oversee your reading, you naturally speak your first impressions out loud (see page 13), which energizes your divining; when others give their interpretations of your situation, the conversation often takes the reading to unexpected places, offering perspectives you may not see when you read alone. And you get to appreciate nature together, to relax and perhaps to talk in ways you wouldn't when indoors. Walking together, feeling the movement of your body and the currents of the wind, is more than physical; it seems to create shifts in your thinking that heighten the way you relate and communicate.

First steps

Reading the land

Landscapes are ever changing. When a wave breaks on the shore or the sky darkens, we're transported into new territory, time and again. That's what makes this type of divination exciting: what you see is precious, fleeting and powerful. You can let your imagination run as quickly as a child's, seeing a man in the moon or a heart in the clouds in an instant.

Landscape readings look at the broader picture rather than life's details; they help draw out themes that are often held at a subconscious level. So, go with a sense of openness and a willingness to feel. An expanse of cliff may feel exciting or daunting. Looking over a beach from a coastal path may offer perspective, or it may evoke a sensation of being distant and vulnerable. Whatever you're feeling, reading the land acts as a magnifier.

You may find that you prefer to be still or that you want to walk slowly, letting your eyes roam into the hills, across the horizon line, into treetops or up to the clouds. Your body tells you when to move and when to stop. Following your feet keeps you in the present moment (the body is always in the present, whereas the mind can be in the past, present or future). If you feel you're tuning out, take your attention to your feet and feel the weight of your body drop. You're rooted. It's then time to immerse yourself in what you see, and let your fertile mind wander, dream and remember.

Reading a beach

Look down on a beach from an elevated position, such as a coastal path, when the tide is out. You may be drawn to:

- **Movement:** cresting waves, the swell of the water
- Reflections in rock pools
- The pattern of shingle on the shore
- Seaweed formations
- Sand dunes and shapes in sand
- The horizon line

Reading fields & grasslands

You may be drawn to:

• **Clumps of wildflowers dotted in fields**

• **Walls and fencing:** intact, broken, weathered
(this can tell you about your personal boundaries)

• **How crops move:** the undulation of corn in the wind

• **Tractor trails in the earth**

• **Fairy rings:** rings or arcs of dead or dark green grass and/
or toadstools; legendary fairy portals. See what the ring
or arc suggests to you as a symbol

Look at the patterns that naturally emerge and let your
mind wander.

Reading from a country hillside

You may be drawn to:

• **Patchworked fields or gardens**

• **Manmade structures:** a town, city, power station or church

• **Road networks and how they intersect**

• **Water:** canals, rivers, lakes

• **Birds in formation**

• **Trees bent from years in the wind**

What do you see? What do you imagine?

Reading the land is a great way to prepare for divination; when you use your imagination, you begin to see structures and natural formations as symbols that your mind naturally begins to interpret.

Seeing rainbows

In Celtic lore the rainbow symbolizes money, fertility and magic. These meanings may originate with the rainbow's appearance after rain, a colourful confirmation from the gods that the land, now watered, will continue to be fertile – and bring prosperity to farmers. The rainbow arc is also said to represent fullness (the Celtic word for rainbow, *kambonemos*, means "curve of the sky"). In terms of magic, in Norse mythology the rainbow connects heaven and earth, representing a path to the afterlife and, more broadly, manifesting through thought – positive thoughts create positive outcomes and what we dream of may become reality – hence the legend of the pot of gold at the rainbow's end. When you see a rainbow, it can signify a new beginning and is a reminder of the beauty in life.

Cloud watching

Cloud watching brings a sense of oneness, that we are part of something other than ourselves. Whatever we go through in life, the sky reminds us that change is constant and we are part of its flow.

It's easier to observe clouds in a relaxed way if you're on a hillside with a view, or you can lie down on the earth if it's dry or look at the clouds' reflections in water. Give yourself time to absorb the formations: huge, low-hanging cumulus, rows of small white puffballs, white streaks or low, grey clouds like waves over the whole sky. See how the clouds drift into shapes and how you naturally give them meaning.

If your mind is too busy, you can see the clouds as your thoughts. Let your mind's running scripts be like the clouds, free to drift away.

When you feel part of the bigger picture, you're ready to cast oracles… and get closer to the natural world.

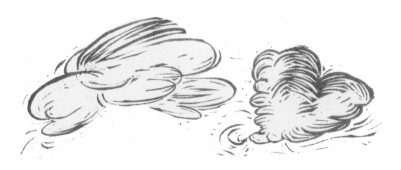

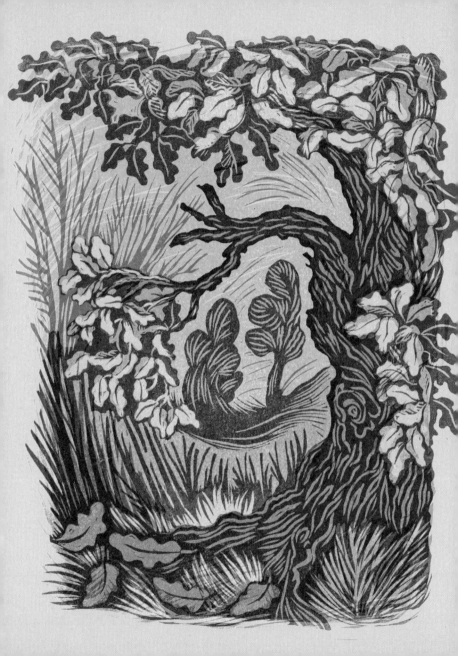

CHAPTER 1

Oracles
of the trees

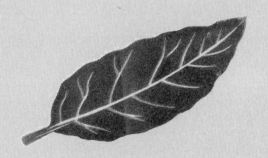

Leaf, bark & branch

As we wander through woodland, silently communing through our senses, the trees are having their own conversations beneath our feet. Via networks of roots and fungi – nature's fibre-optic cables – they relay threats to survival, such as lack of water or disease, so other trees can respond to protect themselves. Through this buried web, trees also feed not just themselves but one another, nurturing their community.

Looking at the tree as a symbol, it's a spiritual connector, bringing together two worlds – earth and sky; a ladder between the visible and invisible, the known and the unknown. Branches can be said to represent heaven, the trunk the earth, while the roots may signify the underworld, the past and the ancestors. The tree, as the tree of life, is a central symbol in many belief systems.

There is a term for tree divination – dendromancy – which applies to divination with the oak and mistletoe, sacred in Druid tradition. In this chapter, you will see that every tree, and every part of the tree, offers an opportunity for answers and for guidance. We can divine by means of the whole tree, or by the bark, branch, trunk or leaves.

When you go among trees – whether ancient woodland, wood pasture, park or orchard – there is no need to be familiar with tree lore or know the names of the trees you encounter (although your meanderings may inspire you to learn more later). It is perfect just to be there, to be present to the trees' living energy and the messages they hold for you.

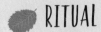 # RITUAL

Forest bathing
Finding the bliss in woodland

Forest bathing, or *shinrin yoku,* is a form of
healing developed in Japan. It's been scientifically
proven to lower blood pressure, boost the immune
system and increase happiness; it's also believed
to enhance intuition – the perfect way to begin
divining in nature.

In practice
Go into the woods and walk very slowly. Feel the
peacefulness, how the internal chatter recedes.
See how the light moves, how the colours of the leaves
flicker, becoming more vivid or soft. Focus just on
what you're taking in, feeling the colours of green,
copper, gold. You may find your hearing becomes
more acute, tuning in to bird calls and birdsong,
or to the tiny hum of faraway traffic. As you drift
further into the woods, notice how your senses track
the changes, the fresh smells and new sounds. You
may find you're walking more slowly and that your
breathing has slowed a little. You may choose to find
a place to sit, or continue your gentle footsteps.

That is all there is to do.

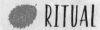

RITUAL

Calling in your tree
Silent communion

When you set out with the intention to divine with trees, approach the woodland in silence. If you're with a friend, don't talk, and put your phone away. Tune in to the sound of your steps, the feel of the wind, the sounds of the branches; as you do this, you become wholly in your body. Your mind makes space for what is to come.

Trust where you walk. Your body, rather than your conscious mind, knows where you need to go and which tree or trees hold a connection for you. Let your feet take you where they want to go. See where you find yourself when you wander freely, with no goal. Your tree will find you.

In practice

When I felt I needed direction, I often used to take myself to the copse in the high field behind our house. Inevitably, I'd find myself guided toward a certain tree. I didn't consciously intend to find it; I just knew I needed to stop and look up rather than walk on. This happened so many times I gave this tree a name. I only needed a few moments here, with my tree – to take a breath or two, close my eyes and tune in. The feeling I had was always calm and uplifting. No one ever approached while

I was there – not one muddy dog gambolling ahead of its owner, nor another solitary walker. My elder tree and I always had these moments alone. I'd eventually walk on and when I got home, mug of tea in hand, I'd know what I needed to do that day. The visit felt like a communion of sound and colour that was to open up new creative possibilities in the hours ahead.

When you've come upon a tree that calls to you, just listen and close your eyes. There's no need to try to do anything. Your senses will act as antennae, picking up signals from your tree.

Many trees have traditional divinatory meanings – if yours is listed on page 31, this may be the message your tree holds for you today. You can also interpret its bark and roots (see pages 34–6), or take fallen twigs and make an oracle (see page 48). But, overall, you can simply form your own connection by being present, opening yourself up to whatever possibilities and messages the connection brings.

Tree & plant messages

The trees listed opposite each correspond to a letter of the primitive Irish Ogham alphabet (named after Ogma, the Irish god of poetry and written language). For divination purposes, each letter was carved into a piece of wood and cast as an oracle. Each letter represents a tree, which was given a divinatory meaning. "The Battle of the Trees", a poem from the medieval Welsh *Book of Taliesin* contributed some of these meanings, for example oak is described as "Stout Guardian of the Door" suggesting the oak is a sacred portal to other realms.

The divinatory meanings opposite will help you build on your intuitive connection with your tree; you may find that the meanings affirm your first impressions, and offer further points for consideration. You can take the messages as advice, such as Birch's meaning of "time for cleansing" suggests a detox, declutter or otherwise making space in your life, or you might read the message as a future prediction – in that a new phase will soon begin.

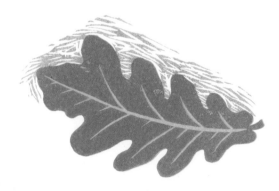

Key to divinatory meanings

When looking up a tree meaning you may be drawn to just one word, or find that all the keywords begin to form a narrative that relate to you.

Birch: beginnings, fertility, creativity; new cycles; time for cleansing, clearing the way ahead

Rowan: balance and endurance; protection from enchantment; healing, psychic work, insight, achievement

Alder: sensitivity, healing, connection with other realms

Willow: community, friendship, co-operation, protection; flexibility, flow, expression (also of grief); creativity

Ash: vision, resilience, co-operation, integration, healing

Hawthorn: challenges (particularly in relationships); confrontation, tests

Oak: spiritual connection, messages from the spirit; wisdom, strength, stability, wealth, growth, success

Holly: responsibility, balance, courage; following dreams

Hazel: divining truth; solutions, inspiration, healing

Apple: choices, love

Vine: sensuality, service, reward

Ivy: ambition, patience, trust, mutual support

Reed: harmony, transformation, self-healing

Blackthorn: restriction, control, external challenges, ingenuity

Elder: change, healing the past, releasing negativity; freedom

Silver fir/pine: priorities, perspective, higher purpose

Gorse/furze: energy, consistency, networks, success

Heather: passion, imagination, luck

Aspen/poplar: self-expression; tension, resistance, protection, decisions

Yew: letting go; milestones; transformation; the afterlife

Ogham names

Below are the Ogham names for each tree, with their initials
and symbols. When you are divining with trees, this initial
can represent guidance from a person with that initial.
They may be living, or in spirit.

Tree	Ogham Name	Letter
Birch	Beith	B and P
Rowan	Luis	L
Alder	Fearn	F
Willow	Saille	S
Ash	Nion	N
Hawthorn	Huath	H
Oak	Duir	D
Holly	Tinne	T
Hazel	Coll	C
Apple	Quert	Q

Tree	Ogham Name	Letter
Vine	Muin	M
Ivy	Gort	G
Reed	Ngétal	NG
Blackthorn	Straif	STR
Elder	Ruis	R
Fir/pine	Ailm	A
Gorse/furze	Onn	O
Heather	Úr	U
Aspen/Poplar	Edad	E
Yew	Idad	I

Further meanings

The additional trees below are not related to Ogham letters, but they have their own divinatory meanings rooted in folklore:

- **Beech:** writing, books, learning; past knowledge; moving ahead; wishes

- **Cedar:** healing, protection, abundance

- **Cherry:** rebirth, love, good fortune, divination

- **Chestnut:** strong foundations, structure, planning; ability to provide

- **Cypress:** sacrifice, healing, protection, endurance, comfort

- **Elm:** inner strength, resilience; the shadow self; intuition

- **Eucalyptus:** healing, protection, help

- **Juniper:** travel, protection, well-being

- **Larch:** identity, connection with the self/soul; life experience and life lessons

- **Laurel:** transformation, divination, ambition

- **Maple:** balance, opportunity, productivity, money. Also love, sweetness of life

- **Olive:** forgiveness, peace, healing, reward, reputation

- **Palm:** peace, attainment, abundance, fertility

- **Redwood:** growth, beauty, longevity, ambition

- **Sycamore:** clear vision, mysticism, strength

RITUAL

Markings in bark
*Find up to three symbols on a tree trunk
and interpret them*

Tree divination, like all the forms of divination in
this book, is an act of creativity, and all the elements
of a tree inform your creative palette.

In practice
Move around and see how the light changes the
appearance of the wood. You might find scratches
and protrusions; bold, freehand shapes that
instantly draw you in; or intricate patterns that
reveal themselves as if by magic as you gaze for a
second or two longer. These marks and indentations
in wood are the messages you need at this moment.

If you are drawn to many markings and feel
overwhelmed, the markings you want to touch are
those you should interpret.

Interpret one, two or three symbols. If you are a novice diviner, work with the starter interpretations on the next page to find insight or make a prediction. For example, if you noticed a clearly defined square, begin with the idea of protection and fairness. The square can be interpreted as reassurance if you've encountered, for example, financial challenges. It may be advice to protect what you own. It may predict an outcome of a present situation – that you will be treated fairly and will have help around you.

To get closer to an interpretation that feels right for you, look closely at the symbol. The more dominant the symbol, the more pressing the message (and potentially, the action needed). Dominant is both literal and figurative. You may consider the square dominant if you feel the greater pull toward it – even if it's small in comparison to other markings on the trunk. So, if your square dominates, the message is to focus on whatever you need that will increase your security.

Reading bark

Letter of the alphabet: concerns a person with that initial

Eye: protection; also feeling observed

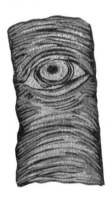

Circle: the completion of a task or a life phase

Radiating circles or arcs: energy and growth; making an impression

Square or rectangle: protection, fairness, security

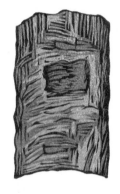

Obvious cavities: count the number. They can signify the areas of life you're focused on now; where your energy is going.

Hatching: intensity; intense thinking, processing that leads to a decision

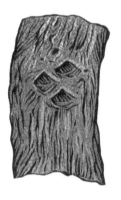

Triangle: ideas, desire, movement, travel

Star: hope, ambition, luck

Runic symbols

The Runic alphabet – a fusion of early Germanic marks and old Italic scripts – has been used for divination and magic since the first century CE. Traditionally, a fruit-bearing bough from a tree such as the oak, apple or yew was cut into little pieces, and each one carved with a symbolic mark. The priest or father of the family would then invoke the gods and consult the runes by casting them over a piece of white cloth. Given the provenance of runes, it feels natural that these angular symbols show themselves on trees, as if reminding us of their heritage. Look for rune markings, and you will find a portal for divination: even the simplest character, Isa – a single vertical line – has meaning.

Here are some runes you might see when walking through trees. The full runic alphabet and their meanings is given overleaf.

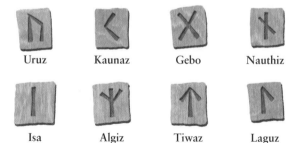

| Uruz | Kaunaz | Gebo | Nauthiz |

| Isa | Algiz | Tiwaz | Laguz |

The Runic alphabet

The 24 runes below and opposite comprise the Elder Futhark – the oldest runes known today. Arranged into three sets of eight ("aett"), the first is named after the god Frey (fertility); the second, Hagalaz, means "hail", or disruption; and the third is named after Tyr, god of war and justice.

Frey's aett

Fehu – F
prosperity, status, reward

Raido – R
journeys, progress,
spiritual path

Uruz – U
strength, healing,
courage, vitality

Kaunaz – K
inner wisdom,
knowledge, guidance

Thurisaz – Th
chaos, resistance,
protection

Gebo – G
gifts, generosity,
partnership, balance

Ansuz – A
inspiration,
communication,
messages

Wunjo – W
blessings, security

Hagalaz's aett

Hagalaz – H
loss or hardship before gain; transformation

Nauthiz – N
restriction, unmet needs, desire

Isa – I (ee as in "even")
reflection, delay, self-protection

Jera – J or Y
time, karma, growth, profit

Eihwaz – Ei (ay as in "day")
cycles, endings, defence

Pertho – P
mysteries, the unknown

Algiz – Z
growth, protection, spiritual connection

Sowelo – S
success, expansion, power

Tyr's aett

Tiwaz – T
tests, justice and the law, guidance

Berkana – B
birth, beginnings, creativity, outcomes

Ehwaz – E
travel, trust, friendship, adaptability

Mannaz – M
decisions, community, identity

Laguz – L
intuition, clairvoyance, emotions, love

Inguz – NG (as in "ing")
protection, love, fertility, development

Othila – O
family, home, stability, ancestors

Dagaz – D
new start, optimism, realizations, change

RITUAL

Reading tree rings
Casting twigs or stones on a cross-section of a felled tree

The number of dark rings on a trunk section denotes the tree's age – one for each year of growth – but you can go a step further. I've found that reading rings, cracks and scars can be a potent way to map present circumstances and divine the potential future. Here are some of the traditional interpretations of the markings you may see, but as ever you will evolve your own:

- **Deep cracks:** decisions, change

- **Minor cracks:** irritation

- **Scars:** challenges, conflicts

- **Widely spaced rings:** happiness, growth

- **Narrow rings:** a slow situation, frustration

In practice

Take three small stones (or three twigs from your Twig Oracle, see page 48). Cup the stones, gently shake them and ask for insight or ask a question. Release the stones onto the end of the fallen tree trunk, then interpret them according to where they fall. For example, if your question was "Will x situation/person be good for me?", using the interpretations given above, the answer would be:

 Two or three stones on cracks and scars: no

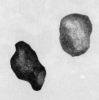 **Two or three stones on wide rings:** yes

Two or three stones on wide and narrow rings: yes, but be patient

All stones on narrow rings: the opportunity may not be worth the effort

RITUAL

Inscribing leaves

Take three leaves to write upon. Let the wind give you a prediction.

This ritual is a form of anemomancy or divination by the wind (*anemos* is the Greek for wind). Traditionally, fig or sycamore leaves were used, hence the alternative term sycomancy, from the Greek *sukon*, or fig.

Think of a question and write the possible responses on each leaf, such as yes, no and not known. You could be more specific – for example, if you're asking about where to live, you might write the potential place names on each leaf. If you're thinking about how to deal with a problem, the actions might be to confront, to step away or to seek advice. To consult the leaves about whom to trust, write each name on a leaf. If it's not easy to write on the leaves (or if you prefer not to), just mentally assign a meaning to each one.

In practice

Take the leaves and place them together on the ground. Wait and set an intention to be open to what is possible.

- If the wind takes the leaves, but one leaf remains. This holds the answer to your question.

- If the wind takes all the leaves, there is no answer to your question yet.

- If two leaves remain, this may answer your question; if they are contradictory, ask at a later date.

- If all the leaves remain, wait. If after a time there's no movement, take your three leaves, hold them up and let them fall to the ground. The leaf that touches the ground first is the answer.

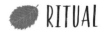 # RITUAL

Leaf messages
Insight from a single found leaf

When I'm running through forests near my home,
part of the circuit turns into an uphill trek. It gets
harder to keep going, the beauty of the woodland
dropping out of my awareness as I struggle ahead.
One time, I found a distraction method that led
to a divination technique I use today. I call it "leaf
focus", and it helped me stay connected with where
I was and why I was running.

Resolving to notice only leaves, I began to see the tiny
serrated edges on some, the star shapes of others, the
shiny greens – I slowed down to take it all in. I felt
wider, able to let go of the goal of getting to the top. It
was enough to just be present. The "leaf focus" soon
became my go-to on uphill runs and meanderings in
parks and forests and, later, a divination practice.

In practice

As you wander or stride out, let leaves become your
focus for a while. Let your gaze fall upon one leaf.
If it's growing on a plant or branch, get closer. If it's
fallen, pick it up, open your palm and feel its energy.

Leaves, as extensions of branches, represent the
"heaven" aspect of the tree. You can see this as a
prediction for yourself, or as a message from your
higher self – your inner spiritual knowing, talking.

Of course, there are botanical names for leaf forms, but to consider these engages thinking; keep it simple and work with the examples below as sparks for intuition.

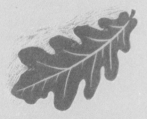

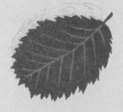

Waved edges:
strength; trust the flow of life

Serrated, soft:
a need for kindness

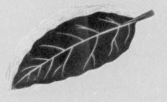

Prickly, sharp:
protection and ambition; taking the lead

Smooth:
creative projects; developing ideas. Pay attention

RITUAL

Guidance from ancestor roots
Connecting with the ancestors

The twisting overlaps of surface roots make patterns and pictures, and offer divinatory messages. Stand close to the trunk, if you can, and look downward. When we look to the roots of a tree for guidance, we are consulting our ancestors.

In practice
First, connect with the tree by placing your palms on the trunk. (If you can't touch the trunk, just stand where you can comfortably see the roots.) Close your eyes, take a breath and take your attention to your palm and fingers: make this a sensory experience. See if you can feel the energy between you. Next, ask your ancestors what you need to know. Then look down to the root formation, still holding the tree trunk. You might want to stand back to see the whole surface network, or feel drawn to one area and focus in on the shapes, patterns and symbols you see there. Next, close your eyes and see what floats in – perhaps a memory in the form of an image, a colour, a knowing, a sound.

Wishing trees

Trees, and particularly the beech, are associated with wisdom and wishes. The origin of wishing trees may be onomatopoeic (wisha-wisha, go the leaves) or its title – "beech" may derive from the Teutonic word meaning book, and the associated symbolism of learning and ancestral wisdom. However, you can choose to be with any tree that calls to you; feeling a connection with the tree helps your wish manifest.

Lie down or sit under a tree and generate your wish. Sense if this is the right wish (if you hear a rustle, for example, you could take this as a "yes"). Take a twig and trace out the words of your wish beneath the tree, beginning with "I wish for..." You don't have to make the words visible, and you can trace one letter on top of another – what matters is your intention to spell out exactly what you desire.

When you have finished, let go of the wish and of any wanting. Ask that you will notice when your wish has been granted and thank the tree.

RITUAL

The twig oracle
Gathering twigs to make a personal oracle

This ritual uses wood that you find on your walks. You can work with any twigs or small branches you find on your travels or in your garden, but they need to be alive – not dead wood – so any recently fallen branches or twigs will be perfect for your oracle. They don't need to come from the same tree. Just choose the twigs or branches that feel right to you. You will need enough wood to cut 30 or so small pieces (see below).

Cutting your oracle twigs

Take your twig or small branch and, using a small knife or secateurs, cut or snip it into pieces 2.5–5cm (1–2in) long. Up close, you'll see the beautiful irregularity of the twig – smooth, knotty, maybe forked at the tip. Go slowly, choosing where to cut, creating shapes as you go. The process of cutting and selecting your runes creates the energy for the oracle. You may see some instant forms: a "y" shape formed by a fork (this might represent "yes" in your oracle); maybe a bud in a fork, which looks like a person – a bud head and two raised arms (so this might be joy, aspiration, enlightenment or, more literally, exercise). You may find a cross shape when you snip off two side shoots from the main branch. Some pieces may be smooth (harmonious, perhaps) and some gnarled, with a texture or pattern that reminds you of something: a knotty problem? Let the possibilities run through your mind as you cut. Move onto a second twig or branch if you need to – aim to have about 20 to 30 pieces to choose from.

Selecting your twigs

Look at each piece from all sides – turn it around, touch it. If one blanks you, spend a little longer, turning it over in your palm. If you still don't respond to it in any way, discard it and move on to the next piece. Don't avoid pieces that elicit a negative or uncomfortable feeling; they're often a trigger for an issue that might need to come up in your oracle reading. When you have 20 to 30 pieces, place them in a small bag, handkerchief or pocket.

Preparing for divination

You have your twigs, so now find a place in nature to cast them. Over time, they can become fragile, so you'll need to find a soft surface – grass, sand or earth that isn't too damp. Spend a minute or two tuning in to your surroundings and sense if it's quiet enough and feels right. If not, move on until you find another sheltered spot.

Casting the twigs: creative interpretations

Ask what you need to know as you gently shake the bag. When you are ready, take a small handful of twigs from the bag, using your left hand (the one associated with fate and intuition). Cup the twigs in your hands, holding them close to the earth, then close your eyes and release them.

Interpreting the twigs

Look at the twigs that have fallen in the centre.
These represent what concerns you now, so focus on
these for the reading.

Begin by looking at the shapes they have made.
In the example here, two twigs form a T shape (i)
and a forked twig has a chunkier piece in its fork (ii).
Two other pieces overlap to form a cross (iii).
All the pieces are touching.

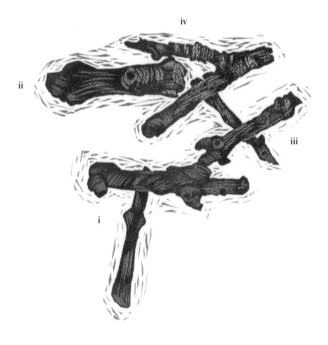

The big twig in the fork (ii) feels heavy, as if the fork is supporting – or birthing – something bigger than itself. (Or, you might feel that the big twig is a huge responsibility, splitting you in two…)

The T shape (i) also feels unbalanced – the lintel is heavy, knotted and supported by a thin, reedy twiglet. Looking at this, you mentally divide up the arrangement. The twigs forming the T might represent relationships and emotions (carrying a burden). The upper area, with its sideways-forked V (iv), represents your outer life – work, money, projects. Do this according to what resonates with you – it may seem better to designate the T as work and the V as home. To decide, see where the imbalance lies in the whole picture. Ask, "Which part of my life is out of balance just now?" and assign those twigs to that area of your life.

Next, there's the cross (iii). It looks as if it's linking the T and V shapes together. It's at an angle, in the shape of a kiss. It could also be interpreted as a warning sign, or simply as a connector in the whole arrangement, asking that you see your situation holistically – in that any action taken in one part of your life affects another. There are myriad ways to interpret and they will change depending on when and where you cast the oracle.

Using a layout: three positions

In this version of the ritual, rather than casting twigs at random, lay your twigs in assigned positions to reveal the past, present and future. This is a traditional three-stage reading, and the meanings assigned to each position can be anything you choose: the situation, the message and the action to take, as shown here; or past, present and future; home, relationships, career; or you might ask about mind, body and spirit.

Gently shake the bag and ask to see what you need to see at this moment and in this place. With your left hand, take out one twig and place it to the left, as shown opposite. Take a second and place it in the centre and a third to the right, as shown. If you are new to divination, see the list on pages 54–5 for possible interpretations according to the twigs' shapes, textures and markings. Work with a piece's physical characteristics first and you'll naturally feel your way toward a symbolic meaning. The suggestions opposite are intended only as prompts; test out each interpretation and modify it so that each twig in your oracle has a meaning that feels right to you.

When you have finished reading the three twigs, choose a final one. This is the "wild card", bringing additional information to the reading.

You can frame the interpretation as advice. For example: if a forked twig means "yes" for you, the advice is to go ahead. A broad, solid twig might suggest hard work – so you may need to assess whether it's worth proceeding. A twig with lots of nodes and buds may guide you to look at all the possibilities before you make your decision.

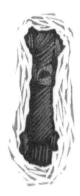
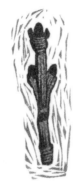
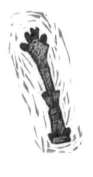

The situation:	**The message:**	**Action to take:**
what concerns you at this moment	insights and influences upon the situation	decisions and guidance

Twig interpretations

Form/texture	Possible interpretation
Broad, smooth	Security, finances, work
Broad, gnarled	Blocks
Smooth, with no nodes or buds	Harmony, inactivity
Smooth, some nodes or buds	Potential, options, travel
Any texture, lots of nodes/buds	Security, finances, work
Twig with lenticels (pinpricks on the bark)	The need to breathe, need for space or time out
"Y" shape (fork)	Support; yes, in answer to a question
Prominent lateral buds	Energy; choices
Flattened lateral buds	Disappointment; no, in answer to a question
A terminal bud (at the tip of the twig)	Innovation, writing

Form/texture	Possible interpretation
A fork with a bud in the cleft	Joy, physical activity, goals
Three prominent buds	Creativity, groups, family
Two prominent buds	Relationships
Peeling bark	Second chances, new from old
Moss	Life, new growth, inaction
Gnarled bark	Difficulties
Lichen	Doubt, hidden issues
Surface cracks (look for letters)	The initial of a person influencing you
A girdle scar (marked rings under a bud)	Change

When you have finished

When you have finished divining, wrap up your twigs and carry them home. If they are damp, leave them indoors overnight to dry out, then place them in a small pouch or bag. You can paint your oracle twigs with clear varnish to preserve them, but I prefer to leave mine in their natural state and cut a new set every year.

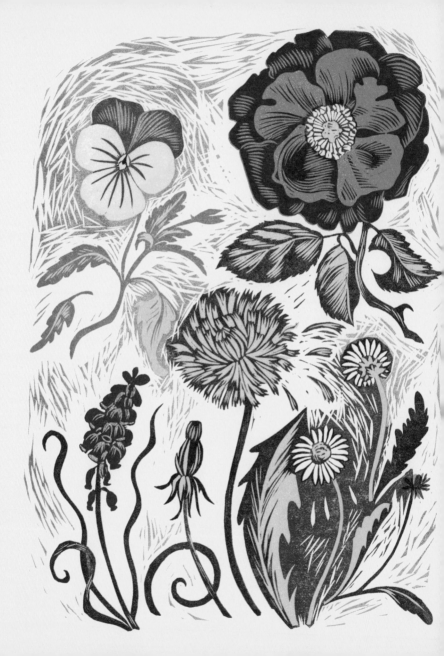

CHAPTER 2

Flower divination

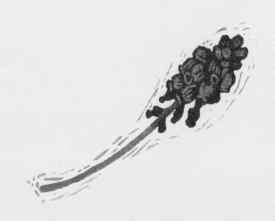

Petal predictions

A flower's beauty and fragrance invite us to open up to the natural world through our senses. This sensory relationship with flowers reconnects with our natural selves – our inner wanderer, chasing colour, petal and scent. When you find yourself smelling the roses or looking at daisies and remembering how you made daisy chains as a child, you're in a floromantic mindset (floromancy, named after Flora, goddess of flowers and springtime, is the art of flower reading). Flowers become symbolic – they're nodding in the breeze, they're almost tiny people. When we connect with a flower to give a reading, we're reading the flower's energy signature, which becomes a conduit for intuition.

Flowers have long been communicators of the heart – the concept has been around for thousands of years. But flower and meaning really came together in the Victorian era with the language of flowers: a lovers' declaration by means of a bouquet. You might say "Alas! My poor heart" with a deep-red carnation, or indicate jealousy by sending a bunch of French marigolds. When divining with flowers, however, we go with our feelings, responding to a flower's texture, shape and colour to feel our way into a reading. Some traditional flower meanings are given in this chapter, but you can combine them as you choose and make your own interpretations.

Take just a flower or two for your oracle work and return it to the earth when you are finished.

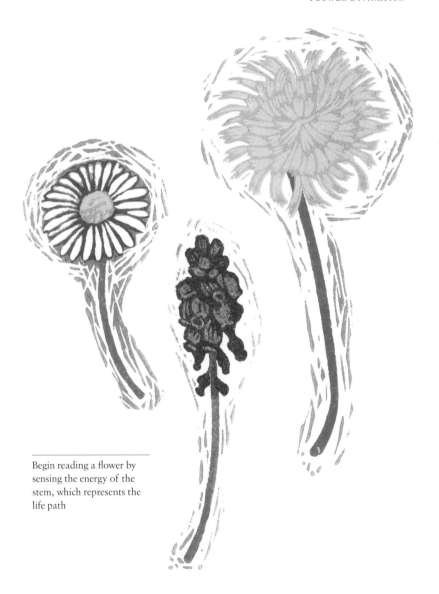

Begin reading a flower by
sensing the energy of the
stem, which represents the
life path

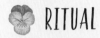

RITUAL

Flower reading:
Read the stem and petals to divine the heart of the matter

Flower divination is a form of psychometry, or reading through touch. To "read" a flower, touch its stem and petals; touch connects you with the flower so a reading can flow. Flowers are associated with emotions, so it's likely your reading will concern something that is heartfelt for you: your life's direction, your purpose, your hopes, your close relationships.

It's helpful to work with a partner for flower reading. If you're new to divination, reading a flower alone can be difficult because we internalize our impressions – with another person you have to speak aloud – and when you speak, you commit (rather than ruminate as to whether what you're getting is "right".) This gives your readings energy and confidence, and, of course, you can enjoy reading for each other, too.

In practice
To read for yourself, choose a flower. To read for a companion, ask them to choose a flower for interpretation. This might be a wildflower you see on a walk or a bloom in your garden. It may be tiny or showy: just be guided towards the flower you want in this moment. (Bear in mind that some flowers are poisonous; go with those you recognize as safe to touch, such as a rose, daisy, buttercup, pansy or tulip.)

To prepare for a reading, take your attention to your solar plexus (between the navel and breastbone). This energy centre – known as a chakra in eastern traditions – is associated with wisdom and energy transformation. Using either hand, hold the flower at the top of the stem. Breathe into your solar plexus and, as you breathe out, visualize white light flowing up to your heart, down your arm, into your fingers and into the flower. See the flower's energy travelling back to you the same way. Do this for a minute or two to set up a connection with the flower. When you become practised, you'll find you do it naturally, almost unconsciously.

Next, look at the flower in profile and from above. Be curious: approach the flower as a unique creation. With your free hand, touch whichever parts you're drawn to. Speak aloud your first impressions. These might be "That purple is intense" or "This petal's about to fall." See your words as the beginning of a story that will lead into another story. For example, petals falling away could signify a situation that has peaked – so there may be a need to release yourself from it, to be prepared for change.

It's easier to read flowers using both hands (one to hold the stem, another to touch). When both hands are occupied, the left brain, which guards and judges our actions, is distracted with a task, so the intuitive right brain can speak.

How to interpret a flower

Begin by examining the proportion of bloom to stem, then see where your reading takes you – the answers or insights you seek may become clear when focusing just on the stem rather than the petals, or vice-versa.

Proportions

The proportions of your flower can tell you what kind of reading you're about to give. A huge bloom on a spindly stem, for example, shows a focus on the mind (the flower head) and what's on show: ideas, relationships and whatever is manifest and current in your life. A thick, furry stem supporting smaller flower heads shows the attention is on the body or the physical world – money, career-building, creating structure and security with an eye to future benefits.

The stem

Representing your life to date, characteristics of the stem – such as bumps, knots and little twists – traditionally signify challenges or life landmarks. These forms may be subtle, so trust your fingertips to find them. Some see the stem as a timeline, like the lifeline on the palm. So, if you're 30 years old and you find a bump about halfway along the stem, this would indicate a difficulty around age 15. However, the key to a rewarding flower reading is trusting what you feel from the flower and working quickly – so you may interpret a mid-stem bump quite differently, such as, "There's an issue here and it's right in the centre of the stem. It's been around for some time now and needs attention."

Other signals

🌿 **Insect crawling on the stem or petals:**
a visitor is coming

🌿 **Offshoots (with or without tiny flowers):**
previous relationships or experiences that you
had to explore, but are not part of your future

🌿 **Leaves:** opportunities; also what protects you

🌿 **Weak or bendy stem:** feelings of fragility; lack of
direction; a need to please others. On a positive
note, this can reveal necessary flexibility, if the
stem is healthy

🌿 **Strong stem:** support, vitality, strong sense of
life purpose

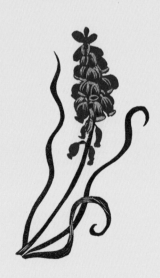

The petals

You can see each prominent petal as a life area, or you can interpret the flower head as a whole (see below).

For life areas, you could choose relationships, money and wellbeing. Or, each petal could represent one aspect of a current challenge. As you interpret, though, you'll sense to which life area or situation each petal relates. For example, you might notice that one petal is discoloured at the edges, which may chime with how you feel about finances. If so, this is your money petal. A petal that's about to come into full bloom, richer with colour than the others, suggests a young situation, such as a new relationship – so this petal may represent love. Take your first impressions of each petal and go with what you see and sense.

To read the flower head:

- **Large, bright, blowsy petals:** openness, readiness for adventure; ambition, communication, a need to be heard and appreciated

- **Small flowers:** diversity; nurturing others, appreciating quality of life rather than holding a singular ambition

- **Single flower, closed or partially open:** a need for privacy; secrets; a situation yet to develop; a need for information

- **Single flower, open:** fulfilment; honesty; "take me as I am"

- **Buds:** what you are creating for the future with your thoughts and actions. The number of buds denotes the number of projects or goals you have in mind.

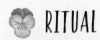

RITUAL

Rose–petal clapping
Divination through sound for an instant answer

This is known as phyllorhodomancy, meaning divination by rose petal. It is believed to have been used by the ancient Greeks for love questions – the rose was sacred to love goddess Aphrodite.

In practice
Take a rose petal. Cup it in your palm and ask your question (one with a yes/no answer). Now take the petal in one hand and quickly clap it onto the other hand. A loud clap gives you a yes answer. A quiet or dull sound means no.

Flower colours and their meanings

For additional guidance, you can also read the flower's
colour and number of petals.

Colour	Meaning
White	Purity, truth; also beginnings
Red	Energy, intensity, passion
Pink	Compassion, love
Orange	Creativity, projects, self-expression
Yellow	Enjoyment and success; health, the home, finances
Purple	Intuition, imagination
Green	Healing, empathy
Blue	Truth, commitment, communication
Cream	Peace
Mottled	Change

Number of petals	Message
One (calla lily)	Courage
Two (sweet pea)	Self-trust
Three (iris)	Finding balance
Four (poppy)	Flexibility
Five (buttercup)	Focus
Six (star of Bethlehem)	Setting boundaries
Seven (rue anemone)	Right action
Eight (clematis)	Knowledge

So, an orange poppy, for example, suggests flexibility with its four petals and creativity with its colour. One interpretation would be a need to be less rigid about a creative project, as there's some negotiating to do.
A yellow buttercup with its five petals asks you to focus on the material aspects of life just now, such as your finances, home or health, to bring happiness.

RITUAL

Petal divination

*Ask love questions; get answers from wind
and water*

As the flower of love, the rose features highly in
the Victorian language of flowers (see page 58) to
communicate happiness, secrecy, shame, jealousy,
pride and truth. Given this variety of meaning,
it's natural that this ritual has traditionally been
practised with rose petals, but you can use any
flowers you choose, provided they are from non-
poisonous plants. If you would prefer not to pick
a flower (unless you're in your own yard or garden),
look for recently fallen flower heads and choose
one to work with for your oracle.

In practice

Before you begin, check that this is the right time
to ask your love question. Take a small stone and
drop it into water. (If you are not near water, see the
alternative technique opposite and skip this step.)
Count the ripples (see Stone & Water Ritual on
page 117). An odd number of ripples is a yes, an
even number is a no.

If the answer is no, leave the divination for another
time. Try rephrasing the question, or ask again in
a few days' time. If it is yes, begin the divination.
Look at the surface of the water to see that it is still;
you may need to wait a moment or two for the wind
to drop, for example. Then close your eyes and take

one petal from the flower head. As you hold the petal, ask a question that begs a yes or no answer. Drop the petal over the water. If the petal floats close to the stone, the answer to your question is yes. If it floats away, the answer is no. If its position seems unclear – it's not really near the stone, but it's not moving far away, either – then the situation is uncertain, so consult the oracle again in a few days.

An alternative technique

If there's no accessible water nearby, simply place your stone on the ground. Then lay a rose petal close to it, asking your question. If the petal stays in position for a minute or two, the answer is yes. If the breeze takes it, the answer is no (see also Inscribing Leaves, page 42).

Whichever technique you use, ask no more than three questions: one question per petal.

Pansy markings

Have you ever looked closely at the number and quality of the lines on a pansy petal? Interpreting the lines or streaks appears to derive from Arthurian legend (and perhaps, the name pansy, from the French pensée, or thought, lent itself rather nicely to divination in the author's imagination). The meanings are as follows:

- **Large, bright, blowsy petals:** openness, readiness for adventure; ambition, communication, a need to be heard and appreciated

- **Small flowers:** diversity; nurturing others, appreciating quality of life rather than holding a singular ambition

- **Single flower, closed or partially open:** a need for privacy; secrets; a situation yet to develop; a need for information

- **Single flower, open:** fulfilment; honesty; "take me as I am"

- **Buds:** what you are creating for the future with your thoughts and actions. The number of buds denotes the number of projects or goals you have in mind.

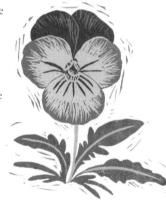

In true fortune-telling tradition, some of the interpretations are woeful – but if you can get beyond this and examine a pansy petal with an open mind, you may just find you intuit your own, brighter meanings.

Flowers that fly

The American poet Robert Frost described butterflies as "Flowers that fly and all but sing". Harbingers of freedom, creativity and happiness – we're attuned to seeing butterflies as positive omens. They're also a symbol of the soul: Psyche, Greek goddess of the soul, is sometimes depicted with butterfly wings, and in folklore a butterfly represents the soul of a departed loved one. Seeing a butterfly soon after a bereavement can be a message that they are passing on into the afterlife.

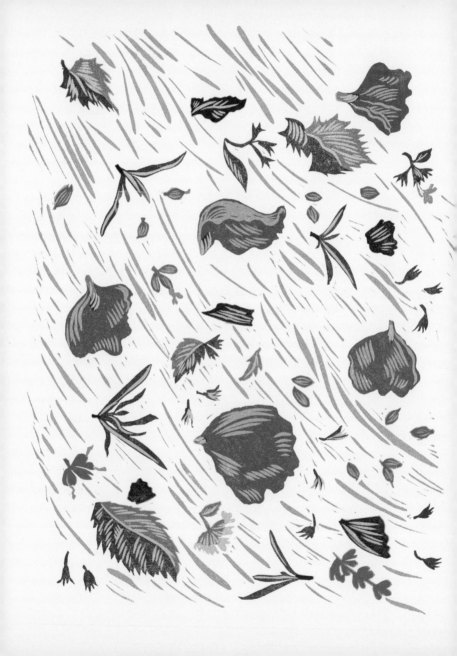

CHAPTER 3

Herb scrying

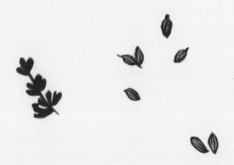

Sensory messengers

Herbs are agents of change, bringing natural healing to the body and mind. Their properties can also help us access a "divinatory mindset" – a feeling of openness and relaxation that helps us become receptive to intuitive messages. Working with herbs heightens the senses, and it's through the senses that we connect with ourselves, with nature and with other realms of consciousness. When we are super-sensory, we are able to read subtle energies: we can divine what is possible now, at this moment in time, and in the future. You can cast oracles with the fragrant herbs you find on your walks and in your garden.

The rituals in this chapter are divided into the four elements of nature: Earth, Air, Water and Fire. We cast herbs onto stone (Earth) or into the air, we float them on water or burn them. The fifth classical element, Spirit, lives in the rituals themselves as the outcome of our readings – the wisdom revealed.

When choosing a herb or herbal mixture to work with, go by scent. Crush a leaf or two and see how the plant's aroma feels: if it's attractive to you and you feel a positive response in your body (pleasure, lightness, a sense of comfort, for example), then that herb is right for your oracles. And bear in mind that you don't need to work with plants traditionally identified as herbs. As you will see, you can gather pine needles, dried petals, crushed leaves or any other safe findings that call to you.

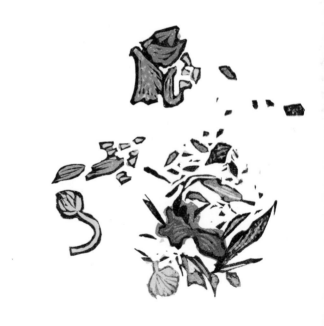

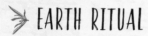

EARTH RITUAL

Herb casting on stone
Read the symbols in scattered herb "tea"

You will need to find a flattish stone or a piece of fallen bark, about the size of your palm or larger.

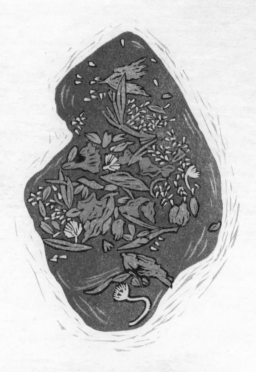

In practice

This ritual is rather like teacup reading, looking for shapes in leaves – so begin by making your "tea". Gather leaves, stem pieces, seeds or sprigs of your chosen herb(s). Use small, light pieces of foliage (lavender, thyme, rosemary or small sage or mint leaves work well). What you gather doesn't need to be an official herb – you can use dried pine needles, scrunched leaves from the forest floor, blown petals, torn grass… Whatever you choose, gather enough to fill the small of your palm. If you have dry material, flake some of it into a dust – smaller particles help create more detailed shapes. Take your time gathering, as the slowness helps you enter a creative, relaxed state in which you stay connected with nature.

Set down your stone or bark in a place that's clear of foliage – damp earth works well, as the tea won't blow away. You'll be reading the tea that falls around the stone or bark, so you need a place where the tea will clearly show, rather than get mixed up with whatever else is on the ground.

Place the tea onto the stone/bark, arranging it so the surface is covered. Next, close your eyes and flick a finger through the tea, once, or blow gently over it. Look at the tea that's fallen around the stone/bark rather than on it. You're looking beyond an object into the space around it, which helps your imagination expand. Be open to what the symbols represent, or ask your question.

Step 1 ritual:
Quick interpretation

Herbs above the stone: the outcome of the situation/answer to the question

Herbs below the stone: thoughts – what's unfolding now

Refer to the common symbols list on pages 84–5 and interpret the symbols you see.

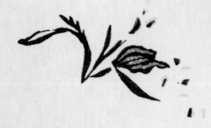

Step 2 ritual:
Elemental reading with the pentagram

Visualize the pentagram over the stone and the surrounding area. This is not as difficult as it may seem – look at the illustration overleaf and relate the areas of tea to the five areas of the pentagram. The pentagram, an ancient symbol of protection, represents the classical elements of nature – from right, clockwise, Water, Fire, Earth and Air, with the fifth element, Spirit, at the top.

The sectors where the tea has mostly fallen show what you have.

The sectors that are empty or sparse show what you lack.

- **Earth:** security, a sense of belonging, safety; finances, the home; the body

- **Air:** thoughts, decisions, ideas and influences; the mind

- **Fire:** creativity, passion, desire, movement, travel; the soul

- **Water:** emotions, love, relationships, intuition; the heart

- **Spirit:** the accumulation of all four elements; outcomes

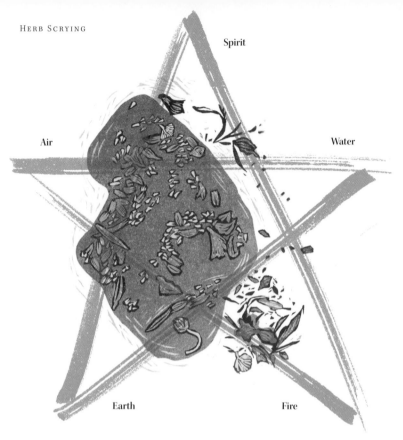

Spirit

Air

Water

Earth

Fire

In the example above, most of the tea has fallen in the Fire and Spirit sectors (remember to look at the tea around the stone, rather than on it). Since most herbs are in the Fire sector, one interpretation is that more is going on internally than externally – some ideas are taking shape, but there's rumination under the surface. This is confirmed by the cradle, or womb symbol: rose petals in a V-shape – something important is being nurtured. While there's a desire to give form to a passion, there's still scattered thinking, shown by the stray tea around it.

In the Spirit sector, we have a single rosemary sprig – it feels as if this person's energies are all going on one thing. There's one piece of mint leaf to the left. As it's touching the stone, it feels like a block: at this time, the person can't see what the outcome may be. Going back to the rosemary, though, it's in the shape of a flower, with petals opening, which symbolizes a wish come true – so it seems that any fears over the outcome are unfounded.

Building the reading

Next, you can look at the herb meanings (see pages 86–7) for a more specific reading. This is where you need to go deep into your intuition and choose the meaning of the herb from the various options that feels right for your reading.

Here's one approach. In the Fire sector, for passion and the soul, we have rose petal, suggesting that you, or the person whom the reading is given, are very attached to something or someone, they love. Given that most of the tea falls in this sector, you are thinking deeply about this situation or person (and may be over-thinking, too). This is confirmed by rosemary in the Spirit sector. Rosemary represents memory, love and intuition – so these thoughts connect somehow with your past. If the reading is about a relationship, it's likely that it concerns a past relationship or someone who is now away from you.

If you are asking about a project at work, you've made the right choice, creatively – using skills you have perfected over time – and may be working with someone from your past, too.

In the Spirit sector we also have mint which carries the meaning of money, so perhaps there's a financial block here – what you are focussing on now may not support you financially yet, and you may be unsure how it will all turn out (the leaf is scrunched, rather than flat, so not wholly visible). Another meaning of mint is education and positive change, so you may be wondering what you can learn from current challenges.

Now, look at the sectors without any tea. Interpret these as what you lack just now, or what are not your priority. Remember, the empty sectors in the example represent:

- ⚘ **Earth:** security, a sense of belonging, safety; finances, the home; the body

- ⚘ **Air:** thoughts, decisions, ideas and influences; the mind

- ⚘ **Water:** emotions, love, relationships, intuition; the heart

So, one reading would be that there's a need for security and emotional support. The lack of Air may indicate a need for intellectual stimulus, or there may be procrastination, as a decision or two are pending.

This reading was given for Helen, who asked about her son who had recently left home to go to University. This was the child Helen had nurtured and thinks of constantly (the rose-petal in the cradle) with the initial G (George, the name of her son) which emerges from the rose. The cradle symbol is also linked with travel. Mint's meaning of education literally relates to George, too, but Helen is unsure if the course he has chosen will get him work when he graduates: this relates to mint's alternative meaning of money, which appears as the potential block in the Spirit sector.

Looking again at the areas of lack – Water, Earth and Air – shows that Helen misses her relationship with her son, a familiar way of living (security) and that she is yet to make decisions about her future. As a single parent, she needs to focus on her own life now and be open to finding a partner, to travelling and moving on to a new life phase.

Common symbols

Your herbs may form one or more of the symbols below.
As you settle your gaze, you may find that additional shapes
emerge. Below are their divinatory meanings:

- ⚜ **Arrow:** challenges, criticism

- ⚜ **Bird:** travel, good news

- ⚜ **Bridge:** journey, risk

- ⚜ **Clouds:** doubt, secrets

- ⚜ **Circle:** success

- ⚜ **Coil:** a problem, confusion

- ⚜ **Coin:** prosperity

- ⚜ **Cradle:** parenting, nurturing, protection, travel

- ⚜ **Cross:** compromises

- ⚜ **Cup:** transformation, emotions, receptiveness

- ⚜ **Eye:** insight, overseeing

- ⚜ **Flag:** protection, authority

- ⚜ **Flower:** a wish come true

- ⚜ **Halo:** guidance, spiritual connection

- ⚜ **Hill:** a test

- ⚜ **Initials:** relate to the name of a place or person

🌾 **Key:** opportunities

🌾 **Ladder:** commitment to goals, growth

🌾 **Leaf:** news, messages

🌾 **Lines:** maps, pathways, direction
Crossed lines: decisions to make (in the future)
At right angles: decisions made (in the past or present)

🌾 **Question mark:** a pending decision

🌾 **Road:** the unknown

🌾 **Star:** luck, wishes granted

🌾 **Scissors:** conflict, arguments

🌾 **Tree:** family, prosperity, spiritual connection

🌾 **Triangle:** success
Downward-pointing: failure, disappointment

🌾 **Wheel:** progress

🌾 **Wings:** protection, guidance, messages from angels
or spirit helpers

Herb meanings

If you come across one or more herbs on your walk, you might like to collect a leaf or two, rub them between your fingers and inhale the aroma before you begin your divination practice. Making a physical connection with the plant, as with the Flower Reading (see page 60), helps your reading flow.

If you would like to do divination work at home, make a cup of lavender, mint or sage tea (or a combination) to sip before you begin your practice. Sage stimulates memory, mint clears the mind and lavender helps you become relaxed and centred. The scent, too, helps heighten your awareness and makes you more sensitive to the signs, symbols and patterns that become available to you during a reading.

Herbs hold messages for you. Note which herbs you're drawn to and see their interpretations, below. You might look at these meanings as what you want, or what you need to focus on now.

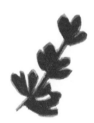

Common interpretations

- ❦ **Anise:** protection, psychic connection, happiness
- ❦ **Basil:** love, luck, loyalty, money
- ❦ **Bay leaf (bay laurel, laurel):** protection, love
- ❦ **Bergamot:** money, balance, energy
- ❦ **Camomile:** peace, luck
- ❦ **Dandelion:** spontaneity, travel
- ❦ **Lavender:** healing, love, peace, trusting intuition
- ❦ **Lemongrass:** releasing negativity, communication
- ❦ **Marjoram:** protection, love, wealth
- ❦ **Mint:** money, education, positive changes
- ❦ **Nettle:** strength, resilience, protection from negative influences
- ❦ **Parsley:** forgiveness and release; also money, luck, travel
- ❦ **Rose:** love, fertility, insight
- ❦ **Rosemary:** intuition, love, remembrance, messages from the past
- ❦ **Sage:** letting go, change, knowledge, decisions, manifesting
- ❦ **St John's wort:** wellbeing, confidence
- ❦ **Thyme:** love, happiness
- ❦ **Wormwood:** mediumship, love, protection
- ❦ **Yarrow:** banishing negativity, confidence, insight

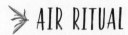

AIR RITUAL

Herb-shaking
Shake herbs to make pictures for interpretation

Take a scarf, a paper plate or a handkerchief. Use
herb tea (see page 86) or gather a simple, or single
herb, and tear or break it into tiny pieces. You may
see a herb on your walk that you're drawn to (see
its meaning on page 77); if it's safe to touch, pick a
sprig or two. Wild mint, for example, is plentiful.
It's associated with asking questions about people
in your life – perfect for oracular work; and its scent
brings mental clarity, too, helping you identify and
interpret the symbols in your reading.

Cup your herb or herb tea in your palm, close your
eyes and set your intention to receive information
from nature. Be open to whatever comes to
you during the reading. You could ask an open
question, such as "What do I need to know about
x situation?" or "What do I need to know about
x person?" Then release the herb onto the surface.

What do you see? Spend a minute looking with a
relaxed gaze. The signs or symbols (see pages 84–5)
represent your present situation. These are the issues
and opportunities facing you now.

Now shake the surface gently so the tea moves
around, forming a new picture. If this is difficult – if
the surface you're using is quite small and the herbs

keep falling into the centre – you can flick the herbs into the air and catch them back on your scarf, handkerchief or plate. What you see now represents what is influencing you. This might be a person, or generally positive or negative symbols that show support or blocks on your path.

Shake the surface one more time. This represents advice – action to take, decisions to make.

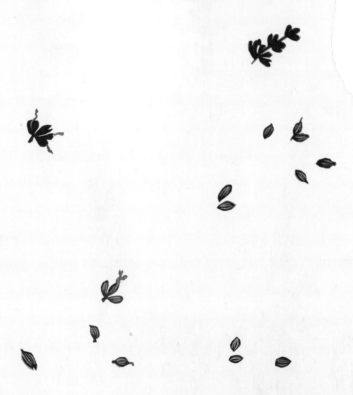

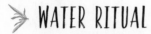 WATER RITUAL

The floating herb oracle
Sprinkle herbs onto water and read the symbols

Gather a single herb or the ingredients for a herb tea
(see page 77). As with the earlier herb rituals, cup
your herbs and set your intention to divine answers
or insight. If you're close to water, you can cast
herbs on the surface and interpret what you see in
three stages:

⚜ **First cast of herbs on water:** the situation now

⚜ **Swirl the water so that the picture changes:**
what's about to happen?

⚜ **Swirl the water again:** what do I need to do,
or be aware of?

You may find that the water moves with the breeze
so you don't need to swirl it. If so, go with the flow –
speak aloud your first impressions, saying what you
see to begin with and interpreting the images. If the
water is still, find a stick or twig and gently swirl.
As the movement of the water slows, the herbs
create a new picture for you to read. If the herbs
disperse and become unreadable, this is not the right
time to consult the oracle. Try again, or in a few
days' time.

Tips: If it's uncomfortable or unsafe to get close enough to the water to see the patterns clearly, take a photograph at each stage on your phone. Later on, you can take your time interpreting the patterns you see.

If you're finding it difficult to read the herbs because the water isn't clear, try placing a piece of paper under the floating herbs and lift it so some of the herbs catch the surface. Interpret what's on the paper.

You can also practise this ritual at home, using a light-coloured or transparent bowl.

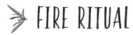 # FIRE RITUAL

Bay-leaf divination
The sound of a burning bay leaf gives you the answer

Divination by burning bay leaves is known as daphnomancy, after the mythological nymph Daphne who was transformed into the first laurel tree by Apollo, god of oracles, truth and healing. Daphnomancy is a form of botanomancy, meaning reading signs in the smoke and ashes of burned leaves and branches. If the smoke rose straight, it meant good fortune; if not, bad news was on the way.

Naturally, practise this ritual only if it is safe to use a naked flame where you are – ideally in your yard or garden, where you can drop the burning leaf onto a plate or damp earth.

In practice

Take a mature bay leaf and hold it to a flame.
Form a question that needs the answer yes or no.
If the leaf crackles, the answer is yes; if it bubbles,
squeaks or is silent, it's a no. The greater the
crackle, the more emphatic the yes.

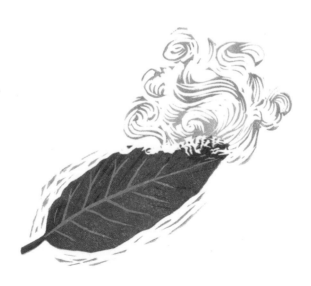

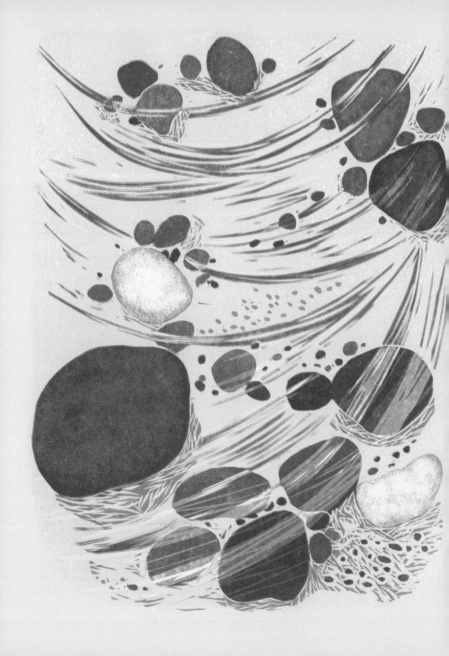

CHAPTER 4

Oracles of stone

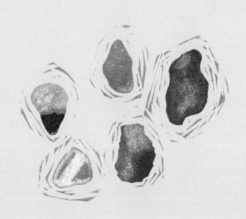

Rocks, pebbles & witch stones

Casting stones is known as cleromancy, or sortilege (from the Latin *sors* for "lot"), the art of throwing or drawing objects for guidance. Divining with stones was practised at Delphi, famed for the legendary Thriae, the three-winged sisters who told the future by means of little "mantic" or prophecy stones.

When you are walking, set out with the intention to find stones you will use for divination. Ask that you find what is right for you today. Pause and look closely. Your treasure may lie on your path: gravel, quartz chips, pebbles. In open fields, countryside or in your garden, hidden stones await. Feel the ground beneath you; lower yourself more closely to the earth. Be impulsive. Let your fingers touch and pick up a stone unthinkingly. The body expresses our unconscious wisdom, the part of us that knows what we need, and it often responds to stimuli before the left brain has time to analyse our choices. We did this freely as children – exploring our surroundings with curiosity, investigating what was immediately in our line of sight. We need to recultivate this habit as adults, too.

It's important to cast your stones in the area in which you harvested them. Through your walking and collecting, you've made a connection to this place, and this enhances divination practice; you're in "respond" mode, reacting to what's around you, becoming immersed. You're out of your analytical left brain and entering the creative mind that's inspired by the natural world. And divination requires intuition, creativity and openness.

Gather your finds in a small bag or your pockets, then find a quiet place to sit and look at them. You may find that you have chosen stones of similar type – those with striation, glitter, speckles, dotted with pinprick holes. Or you may see a variety of shape and form – a rough cuboid, like bitten rock; a sandstone pebble, a shard of flint. You may have chosen shapes like resonate with you, such as hearts, or two fragments that feel as if they go together.

Look at the colour. Are they all similar in tone – dove-grey, sandstone, rust-orange? There are subtle colours in stone. See which contain, for example, pale pinks, yellows, a delicate cast of purple or blue (see the possible interpretations for these colours on page 100). You will need one predominantly white and one black stone, too, for divination, so find these and add them to your collection if they're missing. The black and white stones represent yes and no when you come to cast your stones for a reading, but you can designate them as you choose – white can be no, yes can be black, or vice versa.

Selecting & connecting

Take each stone in turn and hold it. Close your eyes and take a breath. Feel where you are now, in the environment – take your attention to your feet and sense your connection with the earth. Pay attention to how you feel – is there a breeze? How does the air smell? Let your body connect you with the special place you are in, in this moment. Holding one stone, take one deep breath in and out and feel the quality of its energy. Go with your first impression: does it feel peaceful, uplifting, heavy, harsh? Let your intuition guide you toward an association. The key to selection is feeling – if you respond to a stone, you're meant to work with it. If you don't sense any connection, in that you have no strong feeling either way, return that stone to the earth. It's fine to pick up a stone but change your mind when you hold it with the intention to connect.

In total, aim to select nine small pieces that fit into the palm of your hand, including your black stone and your white stone.

When you have your nine, separate the black and white stones and put them to one side. Decide which will mean yes and which will mean no in your readings to come. Then take the remaining seven and go through them again, speaking one word that expresses your instinctive reaction to each stone. Look at the stone as you say this word, as if it's absorbing the words. This will help you remember your association with the stone when you cast it in your oracle – but be open to the possibility that your "feeling meaning" for a stone can change when you're interpreting it in a casting. What you are doing is establishing a baseline, a starting point for you to begin working with stones in divination.

On the following pages are lists of potential meanings for the stones you find, by colour, shape, texture and markings. To decide, for example, on the colour or shape of your stone, look at subtleties and approximations. Unless you find a glowing emerald stone out on a walk, a "green" stone may have a delicate, light-green cast over most of its surface – turn it in the light and see what it shows you. A "triangular" stone will be uneven, irregular and of varying thickness. When you look very closely at a stone, you'll begin to see more – to take in the texture and notice the fine detail and markings.

Naturally, this is only a guide, as what counts is your reaction to a piece when you hold it, look into it and feel it with your fingertips – so take the associations overleaf as starting points, ways to spark a creative response. Choose one category and build the reading from there. For example, the oblong stone (see illustration) means "blocks". As it's two colours, we then get the meaning of "decisions" – so one reading could be, "Making a decision will free up the way ahead." Then bring texture and markings to your interpretation and continue.

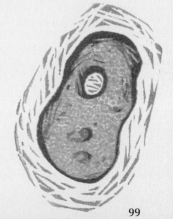

Stone meanings

We assess stones by means of their colour, shape and texture.

Colour

- **Pink:** relationships, love, emotions
- **Red:** new projects, energy, passion; also potential conflict
- **Orange:** creativity
- **Blue:** communication, clarity, success
- **Grey:** the moon; the inner life; what is not outwardly expressed
- **Dark grey:** doubt, hidden issues
- **Purple:** hope, intuition, insight
- **Green:** new life, growth, money
- **Yellow:** the sun; the outer life; what is known and expressed
- **Brown:** home, visitors
- **Mottled/mixed colours:** potential, richness
- **Two colours:** decisions

Shape

- **Oblong:** blocks and challenges
- **Round, oval:** completion, containment, wholeness, harmony, protection
- **Triangular/pyramid:** energy, plans, movement, travel
- **Squarish:** structure, stability, order; foundations

Texture & markings

- **Smooth:** ease, the flow of life, rewards; also a need for calm

- **Rough:** hard knocks, vulnerability, truth

- **Markings:** examine them. Do they remind you of anything? Is there a defined shape or shapes in the stone? With imagination, you might see a wing, a face in profile, clouds, a heart, a spiral, a question mark... let these images lead you to an association that feels right for the stone.

So, before you even begin to cast the stones, the pieces you have chosen are already talking to you.

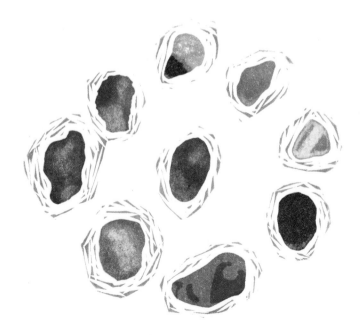

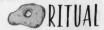 RITUAL

A nine-stone reading
How to cast & interpret stones within a circle

Find a place to cast your oracle. This will be off
the track, off the path – maybe beneath a tree, or
by water. If you're on a beach, cast where the sand
is damp and smooth, or find a dip between sand
dunes. Seek out a sheltered spot, as you'll need to
feel comfortable (it's hard divining in nature if it's
blowing a storm).

Make a circle. Define it with twigs if you're in
woodland or on grass, using pieces you find. If
you're on the beach or if there's snow or you're on
soft earth, use a stick to make the outline, or create
your circle with other stones you find. Sit or crouch
by your circle. If it's uncomfortable to do this, you
can stand – if so, you'll need to make a larger circle,
about double the size. Now formulate a question,
such as "Show me what I need to see now" or
"What life area should I focus on?" .

Take your nine stones and cup them in both hands.
Gently shake them as you close your eyes and ask
your question. When you're ready, release the stones
over the circle.

How to interpret your stones

This is your oracle and there are no rules. When you interpret, you are linking in to your innate wisdom, your higher self that sees your potential and the way a current situation might unfold. It expresses the possibilities available to you at the time of the reading and can reveal challenges to be faced, too.

Step 1: Look at the stones' positions

- **Those that fall outside the circle:** disregard. They're not relevant for your reading today.

- **The anchor stone (see below) and the stones close to it:** what's happening now

- **Those furthest away from you:** the likely outcome, given the present circumstances

- **Those closest to your "yes" stone (either black or white):** where you can make progress; what is favoured

- **Those closest to your "no" stone:** challenges and blocks

Tips: If either your black or your white stone lands outside the circle, continue the reading. If both land outside the circle, cast the stones again.

Step 2: Find your anchor stone

Does one stone command your attention more than others? Close your eyes for a moment, open them and see which stone you immediately look at. This will be your "anchor" stone, the stone with which you begin your reading. What do you sense it might be telling you – looking at it in your circle, does it feel positive or problematic? There may be something in the colour, shape or pattern that reminds you of something else. Take an imaginative leap here: make an association. You could begin with "This reminds me of…", "This looks like…" The stones' patterns, colour, shape and texture act as symbols that link you with memory and intuition.

Here's an example. I've just cast my nine stones, but the piece that stands out is irregular in shape – it's a bitten crescent with a rough yellow-orange surface. This stone feels difficult. I'd rather it weren't so prominent, but there it is. When I chose it for the oracle, it came with a feeling of uncertainty and discomfort; it's come to signify "what is known" and also "truth" and "hard knocks". Whatever stone you're drawn to, accept it – it may not be the prettiest, but it's calling out to you and its purpose is to kick-start the reading.

Next, read your anchor stone in relation to the stone or stones closest to it. They tell you more about the emotion or situation that the anchor stone presents. If one or more stones are touching, read them together. Say the stone touching or closest to the anchor stone is smooth and has a pinkish colouring, meaning love, relationships, emotions. Put this meaning together with the anchor stone meaning, and the two suggest uncertainty or a lack of disclosure about a relationship. In the example, the anchor stone is very close to a small grey stone, representing inner life and the unknown. Next to that is a larger two-colour stone, which means decisions. Put these three stones together and we have an insight – there's a hard truth that needs to come to light, and a decision needs to be made.

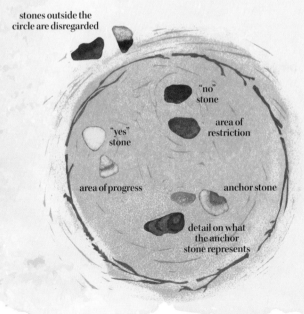

stones outside the circle are disregarded

"no" stone

area of restriction

"yes" stone

area of progress

anchor stone

detail on what the anchor stone represents

A nine-stone reading

The meaning of clusters

Clusters – three or more stones together – can be interpreted as follows:

- **Thoughts:** mental overload; an intense time of processing information, due to studying, for example.

- **A group of people:** perhaps friends or colleagues. Near the "yes" stone, this could mean that a joint venture will be successful.

- **A group of related issues:** one depends upon another, such as money, education and travel.

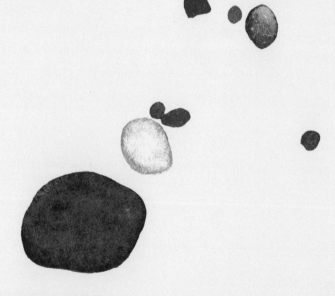

Step 3: See the "future" stones

Notice whether the stones farthest away from you
are clustered (see opposite) or spaced apart. Take
a look at them – observe how they have fallen on
the earth, on the grass or on the sand. They might
have fallen sideways (interpretation: in future, I'll
need to see this situation another way; it's time to
reconsider). They might appear to be sunk into
the ground (a hidden issue that's about to surface).
These are my interpretations, and yours may be very
different, but they show the intuitive leaps you can
take. In the example on page 105, the white "yes"
stone is closest to the triangular stone, so the oracle
is saying "yes" to planning and travel. Under the black
"no" stone is a larger patterned stone that represents
completion and harmony. To sum up: you can't
complete this project or phase successfully unless you
make a decision. When you've done this, you'll have
more freedom.

To make a decision, we can turn to a yes/no reading.

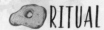 **RITUAL**

A "yes" or "no" stone reading
Casting three stones for an instant answer

To focus on one issue or one person, take the stone that most represents this. Hold it in your palm, and tune in to its energy. Clear the circle of stones and place this stone in the centre of the circle. Next, take the black and white stones, shake them gently and ask a question that requires a yes/no answer. Release the black and white stones over the single stone. Which lands closer to it? If it's your "yes" stone, this says that this issue or person will have a positive influence on the future, while your "no" stone simply says no, so that situation may be better avoided or resolved in some other way.

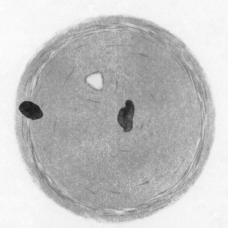

"Yes" stone reading

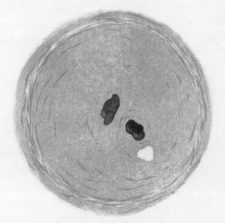

"No" stone reading

Making a spiral to unwind your mind

An ancient sacred symbol, the spiral signifies our journey through life and the cycles of nature. Spirals were carved as a pattern on the entrance stone of the Neolithic passage tomb at Newgrange, Ireland; this may be a solar symbol as, during the winter solstice, light enters the underground chamber through an opening and illuminates the whole space. As this occurs during the season's dimmest days, it's seen as a signifier of new life, the triumph of light and life over darkness.

Creating a spiral can be seen as a meditative practice; focusing purely on what you're doing with your hands, and enjoying the process can help relax your thinking.

To make a spiral, work with small stones you find nearby – you can also intersperse the stones with twigs or leaves. Build it up, setting one stone on top of another in places. Add larger stones to the centre, or decide to have your smallest stone there. The centre of the spiral is seen as the point of connection with all life.

Make your spiral as small or as developed as you wish. Take your time. It's the process that's important here, not the goal: after all, the spiral is never-ending and can never be complete. As you create, you may find you access memories, ideas, questions, passing thoughts. Observe them as they come and go, just as your spiral comes into existence and will disappear in the coming days or weeks, covered by leaves, scattered by the wind.

When you are ready to leave, dedicate your creation. You may offer it back to nature, or make a wish for someone else. You may also ask something for yourself.

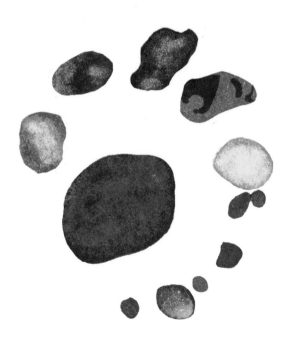

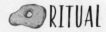 **RITUAL**

The life areas reading
Working with the circle for life focus

If you're unsure about your next steps, this reading can help: its divided circle represents four life areas. When you cast the stones, you're asking which aspect(s) of your life will most benefit from your attention. The stones' presence in one or more sectors acts like a neon sign, saying, "Start with this (relationship, course, debt, strategy)." Taking action around one issue has a ripple effect on the others, so here we're finding a way into the tangle.

To begin, consider four areas of your life. They may be money, career, love and projects; home, travel, friendship and education; children, creativity, wellbeing and new ventures. Whatever seems right to you. Next, divide your circle into four, as shown, and designate each quarter to earth, fire, air and water:

Earth	the body and physical world	money, home, wellness
Fire	passion, energy, creativity	projects, travel, desire
Air	thought	career, education
Water	love, emotions	partners, friends, self, children

Holding all your nine stones in your palms (see page 102), gently shake them and ask, "What do I need to focus on now?" Release the stones over your circle.

Note in which sector(s) the stones fall. Which sector holds the most? Are they evenly distributed? Disregard any stones that fall outside the perimeter.

Air

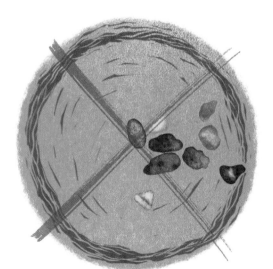

Earth

Fire

Water

In this life areas reading, the majority of stones fall in the Fire sector

113

Interpreting the sectors

Interpret the stones according to where they fall. The more stones in a sector, the more important this life area is in the reading. Then, as with the full stone casting (see page 102), look at shapes and clusters to glean more information about the nature of the events in each sector.

- **Earth sector:** your focus is on the material world: financial gain, working on your home, or body image.

- **Fire sector:** you're looking at what you can create now. A new project may beckon, or it may be time to chase a dream. Travel, adventure and passion.

- **Air sector:** the focus is on strategy. Processing information, perhaps, or there may be a decision to make.

- **Water sector:** the focus is on relationships: deepening a bond, finding space and time for a partner; time with children; time for your own needs. All or most stones in this sector often indicates emotional intensity.

- **If a stone falls right in the centre of the wheel:** deepening your wisdom or perspective on life.

In the illustration, most of the stones appear in the dynamic Fire sector, for creativity, travel and following a passion. The single stone in the Water sector represents emotions, so this may be interpreted as focusing on one relationship. These two life areas are what you need to concentrate on, and the stone in the centre of the wheel reveals that you are discovering new knowledge.

How to end your reading

Take a note of your reading, add the date and/or photograph it. Remove anything you used to create the circle (twigs or stones). Then pick up the stones and return them to the earth, scattering them gently.

If you decide to take your found stones home to add to your divination collection (see Chapter 5), make an exchange: either in the immediate area or out of it, on your return walk, pick up one piece of litter for each found item you take away. If there is nothing to pick up, silently thank the area where you found your stones.

Fast casting

Here are three simple ways to divine with stones. If you're not close to water, opt for fivestones: all you need are five small stones, and you can divine with them wherever you find yourself – sitting under a tree or pausing mid-walk (see page 118–19).

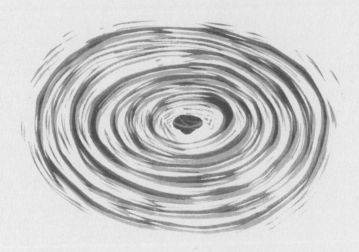

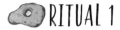RITUAL 1

Stone & water
Interpret the ripples made by stones cast into still water

If you come upon a puddle, a pool on the beach or other still water you can safely reach, find a stone or pebble nearby. Connect with your stone by holding it in your palm and asking for guidance. Now just watch the water's surface and see how it moves according to the air. Look for bubbles and ripples – this is preparation practice for divination, bringing you into the moment. When you are ready, take your stone and drop it into the water. Interpret the ripples, counting them as they emanate from the stone.

- **An odd number of ripples** means the answer to your question is yes.

- **An even number** means no.

For further insight, half-close your eyes and gaze on the water's surface. Then fully close your eyes and let images form. This technique is known as scrying, or divining with reflective surfaces such as water, mirrors and metal.

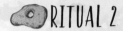

RITUAL 2

Fivestones
Throw five stones for divination

Also known as chuckstones, jackstones, dibs, dabs, tally and knucklebones, this ritual derives from the game of fivestones, which was probably a forerunner of dice. It's believed to have been first played with small knucklebones from sheep; for practical reasons, we use small stones.

In practice
Take five small stones, cup them in your palms and gently shake them as you ask for insight into a situation (if you want to ask a yes/no question, see opposite). Then hold the stones in one hand, toss them into the air and catch as many as you can on the back of the same hand. Put aside those you don't catch. If you need to, repeat until you have one stone remaining. This stone has a message for you. Hold it in the palm of your hand, connecting with the stone's energy (see page 98). You will sense a message as an image, words or an inner knowing. To help your interpretation, you can also refer to the lists of meanings by colour and shape on page 100.

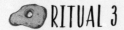 # RITUAL 3

Fivestones – yes or no
Reading odd or even numbers

As in ritual 2, take your five stones in both hands and ask your question. Then hold the stones in one hand and toss them into the air, catching as many as you can on the back of the same hand. If you catch an odd number of stones – one, three or all five – the answer is yes. Two or four stones means no. If you don't catch any, the answer is not yet known. Try again, or in a few days' time.

Found oracles

When you become practised at casting your own stone oracles, you'll begin to see the detail in your surroundings, wherever you wander – whether you have an eye for oracle stones for instant casting or to take home, or you're just enjoying the sense of freedom and wellbeing that the natural world offers. Becoming more used to touching and appreciating the detail in rock, the fossilized markings on beach pebbles, the texture of bark or colour of the earth seems to set us up for what I term "found oracles" – arrangements of stone and/or other natural objects you happen to come across. They may be naturally occurring, such as the way seaweed on the shoreline makes a recognizable shape, or mushrooms cluster in formation around the base of a tree trunk. Alternatively, your oracle may be the detritus of those who were here before you – the ashes of a camp fire, teetering piles of pebbles left over from children's play, imprints in mud. If you notice them, you can divine with them.

Often, there will be a marker that draws your attention:

- A feather or piece of bone

- A brightly coloured leaf

- A pine cone, when you're not in woodland

- A shell, when you're in woodland or fields

- A defined paw print

- Tree roots, prominent above the ground

- Toadstools

You might get an instant "hit" when you first see a found oracle, or you may be unsure what you're seeing, but something in the arrangement sparks curiosity. If this is the case, you may prefer to take a photograph on your phone and interpret the image later, but if you can – and if you're somewhere where you can stop and get close – try to interpret what you see in the moment. Found oracles don't need eons of time for analysis. They are often fleeting messages that relate to you this moment, this day, in this place.

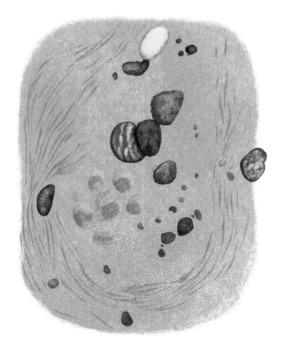

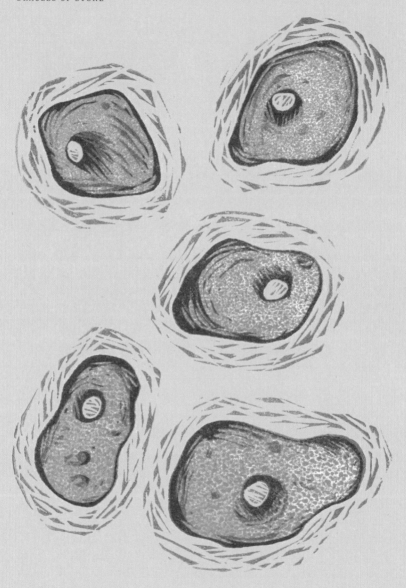

Witch stones

Witch stones are stones that have a hole from one side to the other, so you can see right through them. The hole is created naturally by water pounding the stone, or because the piddock, a clam-like mollusc, has burrowed out part of the rock. Any stone with a naturally occurring through-hole can be considered a witch stone, no matter where the hole occurs (stones with drilled holes are not considered witch stones). True witch stones are thought to be a rarity – perhaps because when you want to find one, you can't. Yet when you're not consciously looking – you may be searching for other natural treasures – they turn up. Then one witch stone leads to another. Others begin to show themselves, and they become easier to find.

Known also as hag stones, adder stones, Odin stones, fairy stones, wish stones and holed or holey stones, they are associated with good fortune, protection, healing, fertility and seeing fairies. Nail a witch stone to your fishing boat for good luck; hang one above your front door and you'll be protected from negative influences. Raise the stone to one eye, look through the hole and you might see fairies and other nature spirits.

Today, witch stones are still considered positively powerful, and you can work with them for divination and wishing.

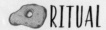 # RITUAL

How to work with witch stones
How to harness the magic of naturally holed stones

Use your witch stone as a portal, as a pendulum or to make a wish. You can also wear or carry a witch stone as a protective amulet.

As a portal
Your witch stone can be a portal to the future. Try this technique in the place that you find your stone – by a river or on the beach, for example. This brings the energy of the location into your reading.

Holding your stone, cover the hole on one side with your finger or thumb. Close your eyes and make a connection with the stone (see page 98).

Ask a question about your future. Let images come into your mind, still keeping one side of the hole covered, as this helps build energy around your question.

When you're ready, uncover the hole and look through the stone. What you need to know will present itself quickly – it may be a word, a meaningful colour, the image of a place or a person, for example. You may find yourself in a future place.

As a divination pendulum

To make a pendulum, thread a length of string through the hole, or use what you have to hand, such as twisted grass or a chain from a necklace you're wearing. Hold the pendulum string between your thumb and index finger.

Find the pendulum's "yes" and "no" positions by asking a yes/no question to which you know the answer. For example, ask, "Is my name [your real name]?" and wait for the pendulum to begin to move. It may move clockwise, anticlockwise or side to side. This is your pendulum's "yes" response. To find the "no" position, give yourself a fictitious name, ask, "Is my name x?" and observe what happens – the pendulum will usually move in the opposite direction.

When you have your positions, keep holding your pendulum until it is still. Take a breath in and out, and ask your question. It will usually respond with a yes or no. If it trembles or doesn't move, ask again in a day or two's time.

Tips: if you're worried you're unintentionally influencing the pendulum movement with your hand, close your eyes while you ask the question and open them when you feel movement.

As a wishing stone

It is said that you can make a wish on a witch stone by taking it in your left hand and rubbing your thumb around the hole, clockwise, all the time making your wish. Repeat every day until your wish comes true.

Witch stones are also associated with moon magic. On a full moon, hold up your witch stone so you can see the moon through it. Make your wish, and trust that it will be granted.

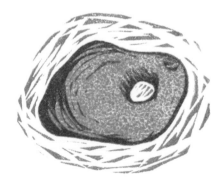

Distant healing with witch stones

Distant, or remote, healing means sending your positive intentions and wishes to a person who is not physically present. It's done through visualization: see the person you want to send healing to, with them standing in a bubble of white light. When you can hold this image in your mind, take your attention to your heart and generate feelings of compassion and care for them, with a request that they be well. When you feel a build-up of energy, open your eyes and send your wishes through the hole of the witch stone – you might imagine this as a stream of pink light flowing from you to them. See the person receiving and benefiting from the wishes you are sending. You can also use this technique to send forgiveness.

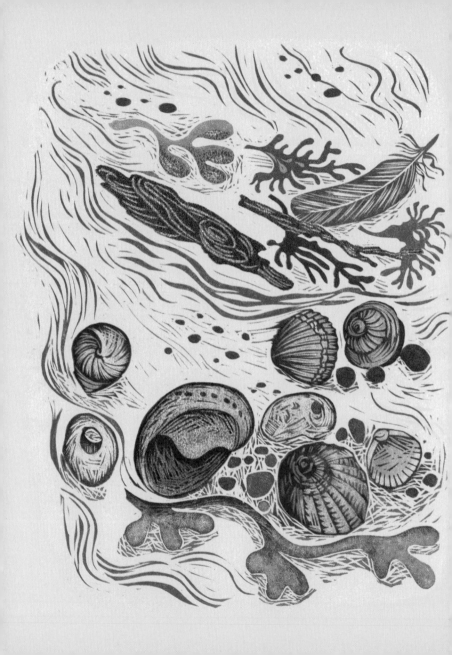

CHAPTER 5

Natural charms

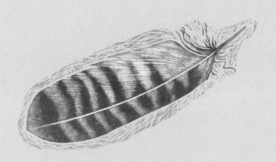

Beach, field & forest

Natural charms are finds from the beach, woodland, fields, your garden or local park. Traditionally, each charm is unique and holds a particular memory or meaning; they're a library of your wanderings. When you scatter them with the intention to divine the past, present and future, they become an oracle, telling your story.

Your charms can be small pebbles, rocks, pieces of bark and twig, shells, seedpods, nutshells and more. You can build your charm oracle by adding trinkets and other memorabilia, too (see Building Your Natural Charm Oracle, page 139).

RITUAL

Making a charm oracle
Collecting beach treasures

To make a starter oracle, collect a minimum of seven pieces on your walk. Seven gives you enough to work with, and it's also the number associated with mystery and wisdom. I've suggested here some pieces you might collect from the beach and how you might interpret them. See page 136 for woodland and field charms.

Beach charms

- A whole shell or shell piece

- A small piece of driftwood

- Sea glass or dried seaweed

- A piece of earthenware

- A smooth pebble

- A rough or pitted pebble

- A small feather

Of course, substitute as you need to. Whatever you find while you're beachcombing will be perfect. If there's no dried seaweed to hand, for example, you might pick up a small pebble you're drawn to and use that instead. If you don't see a piece of water-pummelled pottery, then coal, flint or bone may take its place – or a pebble that's intriguing, and different enough from your smooth or rough samples.

In practice

First, assign a meaning to each charm. As for the Twig Oracle (see page 48), you can hold each one and intuit a meaning: look closely at the colour, feel the texture and see what it suggests to you. Or, as a starting point, you might take these meanings:

- **Shell:** secrets, whispers, the unknown (the shell conceals hidden life)

- **Driftwood:** work, career, paid or unpaid work (wood symbolizes work and growth)

- **Sea glass or seaweed:** relationships, family (water signifies emotions)

- **Earthenware:** creativity, what you are focused on now (pottery is man-made, an expression of creative ideas)

- **Coal:** the past; memories or recent events; skills or lessons learned

- **Bone:** truth, the facts

- **Smooth stone:** positives

- **Rough stone:** challenges, obstacles

- **Feather:** guidance, the higher perspective (a bird is a symbol of spirituality, guidance and peace – see Feather Oracle, page 151)

Next, clear a space in the sand or find a nearby
sheltered, level spot for casting your charms.
You'll need to position yourself so you can cast from
a height roughly equivalent to the length of your
hand, from wrist to fingertip. Any lower, and the
charms will fall together in a central block. If you
go much higher, you may damage the more fragile
shell or pottery.

Take your small feather and put it to one side.
Cup the remaining charms, shake gently, close your
eyes and release them. Stand back a little to look
at the pattern they have made. This reading works
best when you don't ask a question – just be open to
what may come up for you.

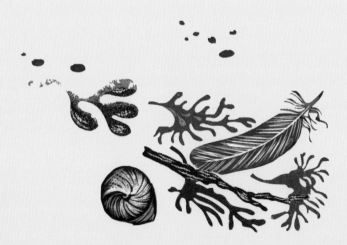

Charm meanings

- **To the left:** what you've dealt with in the past. For example, if the rough stone were here, it would mean that hard times were behind you now.

- **In the central area and above it:** the situation now. For instance, if you had a piece of pottery right below a shell, and the shell seemed to dominate, the message could be that you couldn't see whether a current project would work or not.

- **To the right:** what's next. The wood signifies work, so the message is, "Don't think about what you don't know (the shell). Just do the work."

- **Below the centre:** what supports or blocks you. A smooth pebble here would say that the idea you have is strong. You're building from a position of strength.

- **A charm on its own:** an area of your life that is compartmentalized. It's adrift, unconnected to whatever else is going on (which may be a blessing or a concern, depending on your situation). If sea glass were here, this could say that a relationship was at a distance for now.

Now for the feather. Float the feather above the charms, again from around a hand's height.

- **If it lands near the smooth stone:** a good outcome to the situation in question.

- **If it lands near the rough stone:** a poor outcome.

- **Which other charm is near the feather?** Is the feather touching two charms? This tells you what to pay attention to now, to bolster an already good outcome or to improve a negative one.

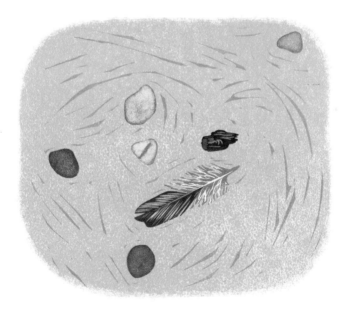

Woodland & field charms

- A nutshell or conker

- A small twig

- A seed pod or flower head

- A smooth stone

- A rough stone

- A small feather

As with the beach charms, work with what you find. If you don't see a nutshell or twig, go with a piece of bark or slate, for example. Whatever you choose, it will reflect your environment in this moment, and this energizes your divination.

- **Nutshell or conker:** as for the seashell – secrets, whispers, the unknown

- **Bark:** work, career, paid or unpaid work (wood symbolizes work and growth)

- **Twig:** relationships, family (water signifies emotions)

- **Seed pod:** creativity, what you are focused on now, hopes

- **Smooth stone:** positives

- **Rough stone:** challenges, obstacles

- **Feather:** guidance, the higher perspective (a bird is a symbol of spirituality, guidance and peace – see Feather Oracle, page 151)

To cast your oracle, find a sheltered, peaceful place. You may like to sit under a tree to enhance your connection with nature.

A quick yes/no charm reading

You'll need a whole shell for this reading, rather than a shell piece. You won't need the feather, so put this to one side. Ask a question that needs a "yes" or "no" answer as you gently shake the shell and other charms in your cupped hands. Cast them onto a soft, level surface. If the shell falls face down, so you can see inside all or part of it, the answer is yes. If it's face up, so you can't see inside, the answer is no. Look at the charms the shell touches or is closest to. This reveals what to do or focus on in a "yes" reading, and what not to do/what to ignore in a "no" reading.

A "no" response to a
relationship question

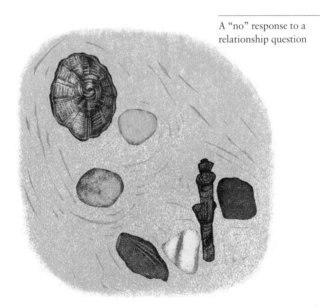

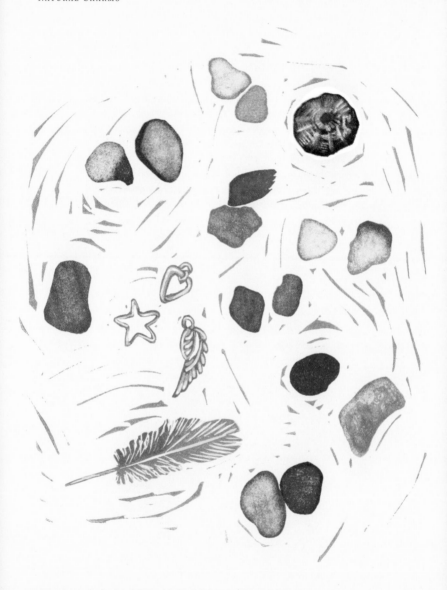

Building your natural charm oracle

Take time to extend your charm collection, adding whatever has meaning for you. You might add decorative pieces, such as single earrings or small pendants, charms from charm bracelets, a crystal or other amulet. These additional charms can give your readings more direction – for example, a heart from an earring next to a piece of bark could tell you that work is the heart of the matter. Further interpretations could be doing the work you love, or even a relationship with someone you work with.

You can bring in dice to give you a timescale in your readings. Complete the reading first, then ask, "When?" and roll two dice. The combined number gives you the month of the year, from March to December. A double 1 means either the first or the second month (January or February). However, timing in divination has its drawbacks – when we have a projected timescale, it's tempting to sit back and wait passively for things to happen rather than taking action. Our decisions change our future every day, so it is best not to hold fast to timings given in any reading. Make a note of any timings, forget about them, then look back a few months on and see how your timing predictions have worked out.

Keep your charms in a box, and ideally do not to allow anyone else to touch them. Over time, the charms become a part of you that you get to explore when you cast them in a reading. You can have as many charms as you wish, and the more you work with your oracle, the more the meanings develop.

Sand divination

Sand divination, or amathomancy, probably dates to the 12th century, with a technique known as Arabian sand divination. The diviner drew four rows of lines in the sand, randomly, then counted the number of lines in each row. A row with an odd number of lines was given one dot in the sand, an even row two dots, which created a column of dots like a domino. Each dot pattern had a meaning, which survives today – from "happiness" to "meeting", "prison" to "dragon's tail".

The beauty of sand reading is that you don't need any tools – just your fingers.

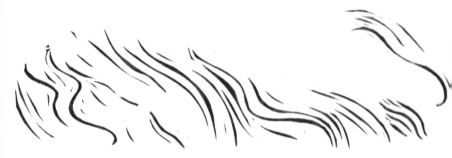

RITUAL

Reading a handful of sand
Seeing symbols in coarse sand

Sitting comfortably, close your eyes and tune in
to the beach – look at the horizon line and take
yourself into the distance, seeing the point at which
the water meets the sky.

In practice
Take a handful of dry sand, the grittier the better
(with very fine sand, it's harder for symbols to
form). Close your eyes and take two or three deep
breaths to centre yourself, ready to divine. Make a
space in your mind, opening up your senses to take
in the wind, the salt smell of the water, the feel of
the sand. Ask the sand to show you what you need
to see about your life in this moment. Holding the
sand in both hands, move to a flat space where
you will be able to see the sand once you release it.
Let go of the sand and scatter it quickly, or let it
run through your fingers. Interpret the shapes and
symbols you see (see Common Symbols in Sand
Readings, page 144).

RITUAL

Sand writing
Write a symbol in damp sand to read for a friend

For this ritual, ask a friend to join you – you will be the diviner for them (it's easier to cast this oracle when you have someone observing, and more so if you feel self-conscious doing it alone). Prepare yourself as for sand throwing on the previous page.

In practice
Ask your companion to silently think of an open question, such as, "What do I need to know now?" It is best they don't speak it aloud – if you know them well, this may influence the outcome.

Take a feather, stick or stalk of sand grass to use as a pointer. If you don't see a pointer nearby, use your finger. Relax your wrist and begin to move it over the surface of the sand. Then feel that the stick is moving of its own accord and let it impress into the sand, so you're making a random pattern. Ask the person you're reading for to respond to the symbol, and offer your intuitive impressions of what it may mean (see Common Symbols in Sand Readings, page 144).

Alternative method
Use a pendulum on dry sand

Make a pendulum with a small stick you find.
Bind it with some sand grass so you can dangle
the stick. If you don't have these to hand, use
a pendulum necklace you're wearing (and even
better a witch stone, if you have one: see page 123).

Make a pile of dry sand. Take a breath and feel
a connection with the sand and your pendulum.
Ask a question, or ask for insight into a certain
situation. Place the tip of the pendulum on the
sand. Then close your eyes and let the pendulum
move through the sand. It may move according to
the wind, but it will usually move without wind,
too (see pendulums, page 125). Open your eyes
when the pendulum has stopped moving, and
interpret the symbols you see, as overleaf.

Common symbols in sand readings

- **Long line:** a journey
- **Circles:** money and love
- **Short line:** visitors
- **A series of short lines:** uncertainty, a need to focus
- **Short, deep line:** a visitor
- **Small crosses:** problems, conflicts
- **Large cross:** if clearly marked, a happy relationship; if not, uncertainty
- **Triangle:** success at work; ideas, expression and focus

- **Square:** a need for stability and protection; a warning to be cautious
- **Heart:** new friends; a new passion in life
- **Bird:** news, travel, messages
- **Mountain:** a big issue; change
- **An initial:** relates to a person or place
- **Y:** yes
- **N:** no

Seashell divination

Shells have long been associated with sound, with communication. There's the conch horn, or seashell trumpet, which is sounded during worship in Hinduism; the folk tradition of listening to a conch shell for the sound of the sea (conchomancy is also the term for divination with seashells); and then there's the shell's appearance. Some shells naturally lend themselves to the idea of listening and speaking – mussels and clams, with their ear-like twin shells; and cowrie shells with their toothed openings, like open mouths. The Yoruba of West Africa cast cowries when consulting the Orishas, or deities, who reply through the patterns of the shells that arise in the reading.

Try the rituals on the following pages with any empty shells you find.

RITUAL

A seashell reading
*Collect three seashells and cast an oracle
on the beach*

You can choose three very different shells, or three
of the same shape. Asking for insight, cast them
onto the sand, where you found them. Casting on
the spot keeps you connected with the earth. See
which ones have fallen face down or face up (face
down means you see the underside of the shell).
Now arrange them in a vertical line, any way you
choose – all face up, all face down or a combination.
This is your starting position for shell reading. The
shells that are face down are "open", because you're
seeing inside the shell. Those that are face up are
"closed", because the underside is hidden.

The top shell represents your external reality – how
you relate with the outside world, how you express
yourself in terms of ideas and conversation just now.

The middle shell represents your inner reality –
what's going on within you: matters of the heart,
your intuition and what's in your subconscious.

The bottom shell represents the physical world
– material concerns, such as work, home, and
practical tasks.

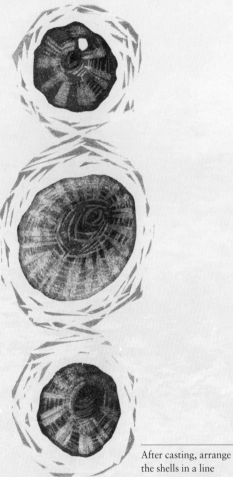

How you relate
to the external
world

Your internal
world

The physical
world

After casting, arrange
the shells in a line

To interpret your shells, think of open ones (face down) as growth and opening up, closed ones (face up) as closed or dormant. Take each shell's position and interpret it in terms of open or closed. For example, if you had your top shell open, your middle shell closed and your bottom shell open, a reading may look like this:

Your growth areas just now are ideas, decision-making and their material expression. A lesser priority is your emotions; there may be an issue that needs privacy. This may suggest that relationships are on hold, or that an existing relationship has become low priority due to greater demands. Given the open quality of ideas (top shell) and work (bottom shell), it's likely you'll make progress now and be able to materialize ideas.

You may, of course, interpret this differently. Being in nature means you often divine in a more spontaneous and less structured way; your reading will also respond to your subtle energy (or that of the person you're reading for) and the vibrations around you (wind, the earth, birds, colour, salt in the air). All these stimuli help attune you to a divinatory way of being in nature.

RITUAL

A "yes" or "no" shell reading

For an immediate answer to a question

Take three seashells (see page 146). Hold them,
ask your question and release them onto the sand.
The result gives you the most likely outcome at this
moment. Given that we create the future with our
decisions, if you repeated the reading again in seven
days, you might get a different answer.

- **Three open shells (face down):** yes

- **Three closed shells (face up):** no

- **Two open, one closed shell:** yes

- **Two closed, one open:** no

Feather divination

Feathers symbolize the element of Air – movement, communication and freedom. In divination, feathers represent messages from heaven. You might relate to this as the collective unconscious, the universe, angels or simply "what is in the air" – influences or currents we sense around us but cannot see. For some, birds and feathers are a calling card from a loved one in spirit (the word auspice is derived from the Latin auspicium, "an observer of birds"). For others, seeing a feather validates a recent decision or a new direction in life.

Feathers often find you; when you're attuned to signs and symbols, they jump into your awareness. If a feather floats toward you, this is an instant message: "You are on the right path." It doesn't need analysis; it's as if you've been tapped on the shoulder and given just the reassurance you need at the right moment.

When you notice a feather that's stationary, you can spend time on an interpretation based on shape, colour and position. We're surrounded by hundreds of potential signs and symbols in natural and urban places, but when an object has your attention, it's because it holds a message for you.

Feathers may come to you in unexpected places – inside your home, on the floor of a shop, on your car windscreen – or there may be no obvious reason for your noticing, other than that you find yourself walking toward it. If you feel pulled toward a feather, follow your body's wisdom and approach it.

RITUAL

Feather oracle
*Interpret feathers you find by position,
form and colour*

Interpret your feather exactly where you find it.
There's no need to pick it up (and depending on
the feather, it may not be appropriate to take it
home). Follow the interpretations below, and take
a photo on your phone so you can do a detailed
interpretation later if you wish.

Step 1: See the colour

Read the meanings for the dominant colours of
your feather – if you see a grey feather with some
yellow, for example, interpret both the yellow and
the grey. If there's more grey than yellow, take
grey as the primary meaning and yellow as the
secondary meaning.

Feather colour meanings

- **White:** angelic or other spiritual guidance, comfort, hope, protection, spirituality. A message from loved one in spirit that they're OK or a message from your angel bringing guidance and protection

- **Black:** protection; also mourning

- **Black and white:** change, decisions, clarity; making the best decision

- **Grey:** peace, neutrality. Also the need to wait before making a choice

- **Grey and white:** peace, acceptance, balance

- **Yellow:** enlightenment, vision, intelligence

- **Brown:** home, security, growth and development from firm foundations

- **Red:** love, passion, energy, strength, determination

- **Red and brown:** protection, fun, happiness

- **Blue:** information; truth, spiritual messages, psychic ability, listening

- **Pink:** friendship, unconditional love

- **Orange:** creativity, motivation; ability to manifest desires

- **Green:** abundance, success, money. Also healing the past

- **Purple:** spirituality, deepening awareness

- **Iridescence:** need for integrity, to see through illusion

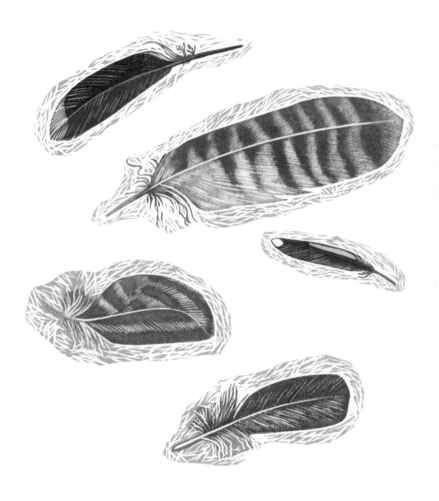

Step 2: See the form

Small, downy feather: a new or young situation

Contour (full) feather: a situation that's fully expressed or known

Step 3: See the position

Tip of feather away from you: what you are manifesting

Tip of feather toward you: external influences

So a black and white feather with its tip pointing toward you shows that a change is coming that may not be your choice. There is no judgment here whether this is positive or negative – it simply affirms the coming situation. A black feather with the tip pointing away from you shows that you're protecting yourself from someone or something; again, this may be a hindrance or a help, depending on your situation.

Feather wishes

Feathers have long been linked with making wishes. Wish upon a feather, the lore goes, and the feather will waft the wish to the gods in the sky.

Take a white feather and wish upon it. Tie it to the top of a twig or small branch you find, then plant the lower part of the stick in the earth. Ask that you will notice how and when the wish is granted, as it may come in a way you don't expect. Say thank you, and continue on your walk.

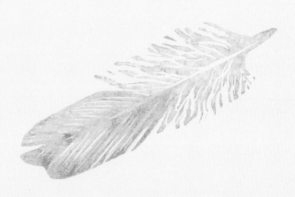

Bibliography

Carroll, John Philip, *An Outline of Roman Divination as Illustrated in the First Decade of Livy's History* (Loyola University, Chicago, 1938)

Dean, Liz, *The Ultimate Guide to Divination: The Beginner's Guide to Using Cards, Crystals, Runes, Palmistry, and More for Insight and Predicting the Future* (Fair Winds, Beverly, 2018)

Grant, Richard, "Do Trees Talk to Each Other?", Smithsonian Magazine. https://www.smithsonianmag.com/science-nature/the-whispering-trees-180968084/ [last retrieved 25 June 2019]

Graves, Robert, *The White Goddess: A Historical Grammar of Poetic Myth* (Faber, London, 1999)

Greenaway, Kate, *The Language of Flowers* (Routledge, London, 1882)

Miller, Thomas, *The Poetical Language of Flowers; Or, the Pilgrimage of Love* (David Bogue, London, 1867)

Acknowledgments

With thanks to Stephanie Jackson and the stellar team at Octopus; to my agent, Chelsey Fox, who helped cultivate the idea for this book; to Michael Young; and last, but certainly not least, to Jean and Eric Dean.

About the author

Liz Dean is the author of 17 books and card decks, including *A Thousand Paths to Mindfulness, The Ultimate Guide to Tarot, The Ultimate Guide to Tarot Spreads, The Ultimate Guide to Divination, Game of Thrones Tarot, The Art of Tarot, The Victorian Steampunk Tarot* and *Switchwords: How to Use One Word to Get What You Want*. She has taught at the Omega Institute, New York; in Perth, Melbourne and Sydney, for the Tarot Guild of Australia; and at the London Tarot Conference and London Tarot Festival.

Her current areas of interest include intuitive symbol reading, divination in nature, poetry, and tarot as creative practice. She lives by the sea in Roker, Sunderland, in northeast England.

www.lizdean.info

Twitter: @lizdeanbooks

Instagram: lizdeanbooks